European Social Policy and Social Work

European Social Policy and Social Work explores shifts in international social policies and how they affect national trends and thus the context for social work practice.

The book discusses international and national social work strategies and practice and investigates the responsibilities for social welfare held by the state, the market and civil society. Van Ewijk then elaborates a new concept of citizenship-based social work which supports and encourages self-responsibility, social responsibility and the implementation of social rights. The main themes covered are:

- International social policy and social work
- From welfare to workfare
- Citizenship
- Essentials of citizenship-based social work
- Community policy and community work
- Social work and alternative areas of activity such as youth care and social care.

Integrating different roots and social professions in an overarching new concept, this book looks particularly at European Union countries. Van Ewijk examines debates regarding social work as an internationally recognized profession and science.

This book is suitable for social work students, academics and professionals with an interest in social policy and international social work.

Hans van Ewijk is Professor of Social Policy and Social Work and Chair of the Research Centre for Social Innovation at Utrecht University of Applied Sciences, the Netherlands. He was recently appointed as Endowed Professor at the University for Humanistics at Utrecht for the Chair of Social Work Theory and is also Visiting Professor at Tartu University, Estonia. He is a former president of the International Council on Social Welfare Europe.

European Social Policy and Social Work

Citizenship-based social work

Hans van Ewijk

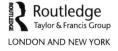
Routledge
Taylor & Francis Group

LONDON AND NEW YORK

First published 2010
by Routledge
2 Park Square, Milton Park, Abingdon, Oxon, OX14 4RN

Simultaneously published in the USA and Canada
by Routledge
711 Third Avenue, New York, NY 10017

Routledge is an imprint of the Taylor & Francis Group, an informa business

© 2010 Hans van Ewijk

Typeset in Times New Roman
by Keystroke, Tettenhall, Wolverhampton

British Library Cataloguing in Publication Data
A catalogue record for this book is available from the British Library

Library of Congress Cataloging-in-Publication Data
Ewijk, Hans van.
  European social policy and social work : citizenship-based social work / Hans van Ewijk.
    p. cm.
    1. European Union countries–Social policy. 2. Social service–European Union countries.
    I. Title.
    HN373.5.E95 2009
    361.3094–dc22
    2009011800

ISBN13: 978–0–415–54521–1 (hbk)
ISBN13: 978–0–415–54523–5 (pbk)
ISBN13: 978–0–203–86992–5 (ebk)

Contents

Illustrations

Figures

Tables

Introduction

What the book is about

European social policy and social work: citizenship-based social work explores the transformation of European states into activating welfare states and their impact on social work. The 'activating welfare state' is based on a balanced mix of productivity, participation, cohesion and knowledge. It enables and endorses citizenship, civil society and the market within a steering and regulating framework, set by international, national, regional and local governments. Social work should adapt to this transformation process by repositioning itself, by redefining its concepts and strategies, and by reconsidering its methods and approaches. I define this redirection process within social work as 'citizenship-based social work'. 'Social work' refers to a common field of social action, social theories and social work research. It is based on an international shared social work body of knowledge. 'Citizenship' or activating citizenship connects to the idea 'to put citizens first' (Stevens and Sullivan 2001). It is up to citizens as residents, as users, as political beings to define social problems and to co-operate in improving social contexts, in supporting vulnerable people and critical situations and to influence political decision-making processes. The main task of social professionals – like social workers, community workers, social care workers, social pedagogues, youth workers, social and creative therapists – is to enable and support people in critical situations to keep control of their own needs, problems and interventions. Social professionals' primary task is to support the social environment – family, friends, communities, schools, workplace – in creating better social conditions and supporting vulnerable people and vulnerable neighbourhoods. Social professionals start from the context people are in, looking from there to who could contribute and improve it and, if needed, takes action to address relevant actors, to bring them together and to implement social actions and social support.

Citizenship-based social work is embedded in the transformation to the activating welfare state and directs enabling citizens to take their individual and social responsibility, based on a strong system of civil, political and social rights. It recognizes citizenship as contextual, relative and relational, according to the principle of each citizen to their own capabilities and capacities. Citizenship is not an exclusive standard but an inclusive one. It is not a pure individual enterprise but refers to a society that includes each citizen with their own talents, characteristics and peculiarities.

This book does not provide a full social work overview. It is more of a redirection of social work in the framework of transformation of our societies. It discusses the perspectives, basic assumptions and dominant concepts in social work and seeks to connect to social policy. It does not fit easily into Malcolm Payne's triangle dividing social work into 'reflexive-therapeutic', 'individualist-reformist' and 'socialist-collectivist' (Payne 2005, p. 10). This book is definitely not in the reflexive-therapeutic corner. This does not mean that this branch of social work is not relevant, far from it, but it is not the perspective here. The book is neither in the socialist-collectivist corner. As I will argue in this book, we are moving from a social policy debate focused on national systems and socio-economic perspectives to a much more social-cultural focus, asking for contextual and local actions and policies aiming at concepts such as safety, livability, social capital, social competences, social cohesion, participation and integration. Maybe we should transfer Payne's triangle into a square, with a dedicated corner for contextual transformational social work, being different from 'individualist-reformist', Payne's third and not highly valued corner within the social work discourse. Citizenship-based social work is contextual and tries to transform situations people are in. In my opinion, it is different from 'individualist' because it includes social environments and communities, and different from reformist because it is built upon the idea of a continuing transformation of societies and communities.

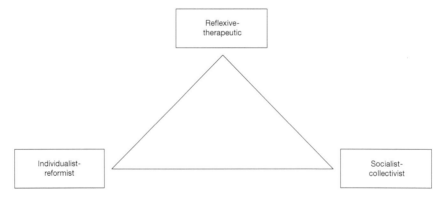

Figure 0.1 Payne triangle (Payne 2005: 10).

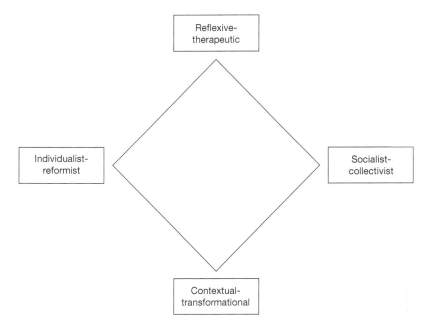

Figure 0.2 Social work square.

For whom is the book useful?

European social policy and social work: citizenship-based social work has been developed as a course for Masters students, building upon a certain knowledge of theories and practices in social policy and social work. Therefore, Masters students and advanced undergraduate students in social work and social policy are the main target group. However, the publication is aimed also at senior social workers and social policy makers who want to deepen and broaden their knowledge and insights into current developments in (European) social policy and social work. To support students in dealing with the substance, some questions and assignments have been added at the end of each chapter.

What the chapters are about

Chapter 1 is an introductory chapter which embeds regional, national and local social policy and social work in the shared framework of international social work. International social work stands for a common field of action and an international body of knowledge of practice and theories, its impact on national and local social work and being part of an international community. The chapter starts with discussing the concepts of international social work and globalization and focuses in its second part on the process of regionalization in Europe: the European Union, the Council of Europe and the Bologna Declaration.

Chapter 2 outlines the transformation process we are all in, characterized by privatization, civil society, localization and integration, summarized in a reflection on the shift from a socio-economic thinking to a more social-cultural approach. I intend to focus on the European Union concept of the activating welfare state as an alternative for the Anglo-Saxon workfare state. The so-called European model integrates cohesion and a decent level of social security into the activating perspective. In the European transformation process, participation should be balanced between participating in work, in care, in communities, in civil society and in the political arena.

Chapter 3 reflects on the concepts of citizenship and civil society. Starting with Marshall's civil, political and social rights and endorsing Lister's idea of 'lived citizenship'. Citizenship is not an exclusive standard but a societal assignment to enable each citizen to live up to social citizenship – individual and social responsibility based on social rights and duties – to his or her own capacities and capabilities. 'Societal assignments' imply the co-operation between the public sector, civil society and the market as the essential actors to guarantee citizenship to all people.

Chapter 4 clarifies the concept of social work, investigating the meanings, the roots, the discourses and the professions and explores the impact of the transformation process on the positions, core tasks, basic methodology and competences of social professionals. It defines citizenship-based social work as a field of action, knowledge and research, aiming at integration of all citizens, and supporting and encouraging self-responsibility, social responsibility and the implementation of social rights and duties.

Chapter 5 deals with an often neglected field in social work. This is considered first, because citizenship-based social work is embedded firmly in community policy and practice. The chapter sketches the history of the community idea and the recent interest in community policies and goes on to discuss the essence and importance of local social policy making, aiming at communities and contexts, and moves on to community work, its roots and definition as the contribution from social professionals, together with and geared to the local citizens, in strengthening social cohesion, social capital and social competences of communities and their residents. From there, we discuss the roles, tasks and methods in community work.

Chapter 6 explores youth work, youth care, long term care, and fighting exclusion and poverty. It is based on the idea of the main 'zones' in local social policies. Youth work and youth care are connected to the assignment to create a challenging, protective and participative world for children and young people to grow up in. It positions social professionals in youth work, child care, youth care and in the role of supporting and enabling an empowering environment. Long term care starts from the interconnection between health, housing, care, welfare and an accessible environment. It focuses on the most vulnerable citizens and the role of social professionals in delivering care and support, and in creating accessible and supportive environments. Social work, exclusion and poverty focuses on fighting exclusion and oppression. On the one side we find social case workers intervening in the complex situations people are in and vulnerable people who need 'care and social management'. On the other side we find social professionals involved in strategies to fight against exclusion, oppression and poverty by empowerment, by supporting emancipating processes and by trying to change or at least adjust social systems, such as education, the labour market, social security, transport, urban planning, health and housing.

Chapter 7 provides an overview of economic and socio-cultural discourses on migration, from a melting pot to transnational regionalization. In its second part we discuss intercultural social work, its competences, the need for knowledge and the challenges for social work and social work education.

Chapter 8 discusses the profession, standards and ethics, the body of knowledge, and social work research. It recognizes social work as a science because it encompasses a huge body of knowledge on theories, practices and methods, connected to policy-making processes and integrating different scientific disciplines. The lack of an overarching theory is hardly problematic because modern sciences are lacking paradigms and are all in a dis-consensus discourse. To study intervening and enabling theories, strategies and methods in the field of social behaviour and social relationships means studying a highly complex reality, needing a strong scientific base, all the more so, because social services are one of the biggest sectors in Europe and one of the fast growing ones, as well.

The Utrecht-Tartu connection

I hope *European social policy and social work: citizenship-based social work* contributes to the essential debate about the direction, strategy and concepts in social work. Social work includes all kinds of social practices and social professions. In this book, social work is a much wider concept as in the traditional Anglo-Saxon approach with its strongly public sector-connected social case worker and the focus on short interventions. In this sense, the concepts of this book are based more on the social work in the Nordic and Western continental welfare states but challenging the UK, Southern Europe and post-socialist states. This book originated from Masters courses at Tartu University in Estonia. Students in this small Baltic country – with no experience of a welfare state but a former Soviet state and a highly chaotic period in the early 1990s – were highly interested in this citizenship and community-based social work approach and thanks to them and my colleagues at the Institute of Sociology and Social Policy (excluding social work in the title), I felt encouraged to submit the course book to Routledge for publication. The other important source for creating this concept and writing the book was the Utrecht University of Applied Sciences, changing itself from a teaching university into a research university of applied sciences, and setting up a Research Centre for Social Innovation. At Utrecht University/HU there are over 3,000 undergraduate social work students but no tradition of research degrees. The Netherlands was one of the first countries in the world to establish social work education and for many decades was one of the leading European countries in expanding and exploring social theories, partly based in the old university departments and faculties in social pedagogy and Dutch attempts to establish new social work-related sciences. Those 'old university-based embedments' disappeared in the 1980s and 1990s and undergraduate social work was only studied at the 'hogescholen'. One of the ambitions of our social innovation research centre is to create a new Dutch tradition in science and research embedded in the expanding process of international social work and so we started Masters courses in social work and pedagogy and developed the research centre in a few years to one with nine professors, 17 PhD students (teachers from the faculty) and approximately 80 senior teachers/researchers and many undergraduate and Masters students.

It would be very helpful if readers of this book could send me their comments.

Hans van Ewijk
Professor in (International) Social Policy and Social Work HU and UT
Chair Research Centre Social Innovation, Utrecht University
of Applied Sciences / HU

Hans.vanewijk@hu.nl
Utrech/Tartu, 2009

1 International social work and international social policy

Introduction

The first part of this chapter places social work in the broader framework of international social work and social policy. In the first section we explain what 'international social work' is. It has developed from a rather precise and specified area – working in international agencies – to a much broader concept. International social work and international social policy are both part of the globalization process. The second part of this chapter concentrates on the so-called regionalization in Europe, the process to strengthen co-operation between nation states in a certain region. The strongest and most striking regionalization process is the creation and enlargement of the European Union. A second regionalization is found in the Council of Europe embracing all European countries. A third regionalization used to be the Soviet bloc. However, nowadays, the Russian Federation is regarded more as a nation state and not a regional co-operation of independent countries. An important impact on the field of higher education, and therefore essential for social work, has been the Bologna Declaration in 1999.

Different meanings of international social work and social policy

International social work and social policy is a recognized specific field in social work with its own discourse, publications and even a specific journal, *International Social Work*. At US universities international social work is an obligatory course for all Masters students. In European countries it is usually an individual course or integrated in other subjects of the social work curriculum. Let us first look a little closer at the different interpretations of international social work.

Cross-border social work

Originally international social work stood for social work in international agencies, like the Red Cross, UNICEF or Amnesty International. It was assumed that social workers needed a specific training for social work in human relief, community building, advocacy, lobbying and international relationships. A second branch was more of a policy making one in international bodies like the United Nations,

UNESCO, the European Union or the Council of Europe. A third area encompassed the possibility of becoming a social worker in another country. For that reason, international social work associations attempted to create a common understanding of the social professions. In the European region, within the framework of the Bologna Declaration, agreements have been made about interchanges based on recognized profiles and trainings (1999). Social work across the borders occurs mostly between countries with the same native language because social work is a highly sensitive area as far as language and culture are concerned (Xu 2006).

Comparative studies

In comparative studies, practices, contexts, processes and theories from different countries are under investigation. It creates opportunities for mutual learning processes and for bench marking processes. Comparative studies are often carried out in networks of universities or in mutual agreements between different countries. International agencies, such as OECD (Organization for Economic Co-operation and Development) and UNRISD (United Nations Research Institute for Social Development) support, carry out and disseminate international studies and research. In recent decades the European Union has authorized a considerable number of comparative studies on issues like social care, employment, citizenship, equal opportunities and youth mobility. An important agency is EU-Research, its commissioner and framework. Apart from this, each EU directorate (ministry) has its own research funding. In higher education, research co-operation is endorsed within the framework of the Life Long Learning Programme. A specific method within the EU is the Open Method of Coordination (OMC), implying an ongoing discourse on, and monitoring of, developments in a certain field in the different EU member states. Related to OMC are the National Action Plans (NAP). In a National Action Plan, countries account for the national policy and national achievements in a certain sector, for example, the social sector on the issue of social inclusion. This exchanging of information and knowledge, and comparing (social) development in different areas creates a mutual learning process in the EU states and sectors. The effect is that countries are creating a common discourse and mutual understanding (Tomka 2003).

Advocacy

Here, international social work is in the perspective of advocacy for social justice and fighting poverty. Social work has always been closely related to religious and socialist or social democrat ideologies fighting for the most excluded and advocating the interests of the poor, the marginal, and excluded people. Nowadays, representatives from the South are reminding Western social workers of this tradition. In their eyes, social workers are hiding too much from the international community and are failing to champion the rights of the poor. International social work has to move from its Eurocentric and ethnocentric milieu (Ahmadi 2003).

In international bodies like ECOSOC (UN), the EU-ECOSOS and the Platform of European Social NGOs, advocacy for the excluded is seen as an important way of influencing global and European politics.

Cross-cultural and intercultural competences and awareness

The growing mobility of people creates new challenges to modern societies. People should live up to a greater diversity and therefore intercultural competences and global awareness are needed (Xu 2006). Diversity asks for social workers to understand people from different national and ethnic backgrounds and to strengthen their social and cultural competences. Intercultural social work is a fast growing body of knowledge and factual practice all over Europe (see Chapter 7).

International transfer of social work knowledge

Here we find a much broader concept of international social work. It is about transfer from knowledge of, first, practices, methods and experiences, second, theories and concepts, and third, social policies and social work policies. It refers to a common international body of knowledge and an international recognized field of action. Recently, international social work has been defined more broadly as 'a professional practice that crosses national boundaries, and relies on contacts and exchanges between countries' (Xu 2006). As early as 1928 social services, social professionals and social educators met in Paris and established the International Council on Social Welfare/ICSW. In the 1950s the International Federation of Social Workers/IFSW and the International Association of Schools of Social Work/IASSW broke away from ICSW and became independent international organizations (Lyons 1999, Healy 2001, Lyons *et al.* 2006). Those different networks aimed to exchange knowledge, develop an international understanding of social welfare and social work and they stood for professional expertise on the global and regional level. Recently, those three still existing international networks decided to co-operate more intensively on the global level. In Europe they created a European Umbrella, ENSACT, for civil society, social workers and social educators, including seven European networks. ENSACT voices the professional expertise in Europe and aims to expand and deepen social work's body of knowledge. Organizing conferences and expert meetings was the first action in creating an international social work body of knowledge. Nowadays, there is a huge pile of publications on (international) social work, a long list of international journals and many international networks dedicated to all kind of social work issues and fields of activities (Healy 2001, Irving and Payne 2005, Xu 2006).

The international community

Social workers all over the world have one thing in common: they look at people and societies from the social perspective. That is different from doctors looking from the health perspective or lawyers interpreting reality from the law or economists perceiving societies and people from the economic viewpoint. Social workers are value based with social justice as their core value and they want to support people to improve their situations, their relationships, their social and cultural competencies, and their behaviour. This recognition of the social perspective, the social profession, the social practice and theory, binds social workers all over the world together into one of the biggest virtual communities.

Conclusion

All those aspects of international social work belong to its own domain. For me, international social work stands for a common field of action and an international body of knowledge of practice and theories, their impact on national and local social work and belonging to an international community. It includes cross-cultural awareness, advocacy, and transfer of knowledge, working abroad and comparative studies. International social work is essential for social professionals in profiling social work as an important mean in getting social policies to work. Social professionals have to overcome narrowing their scope to merely dealing with clients in local situations. They should be able to function and reflect in an international and cross-cultural context.

Globalization

Perspectives

Globalization is a complex and contested concept provoking fierce debates and can be viewed as a process that is going on (a fact), or as a deliberate strategy or a combination of both. We distinguish the next interpretations:

1   Globalization is often perceived as an economic strategy as a trend to free trade or an open market. In that respect it is contested as well because it is regarded as an injustice to poorer countries. Those countries lack capital and human resources to compete with the wealthy and well developed countries, and therefore they are losers before competition starts. Anti-globalists are fighting for a more equal level playing field or even oppose fully an open market strategy.
2   Globalization is also concerned with a compression of time and place. People can travel around the world in a day and by the internet in less than a second. Even in the most remote places in this world people can connect to other people in other continents. News is spread all over the world in a few seconds. Therefore we all live to a great extent in a common world.
3   Globalization can be seen and felt as a McDonaldization as well. We find the same labels, shops, restaurants and music everywhere. Marcuse once analysed it as getting into a one-dimensional world (1964) as a world dominated by a mass culture, leaving out historical diversities and a great belief in progress as getting more individual affluence.

4   Another perspective on globalization is the development of a more social world. A global discourse on social policies based on fundamental rights and social justice is ongoing. The UN and nearly all the nations of the world have accepted a number of treaties and conventions on human and social rights. However, a great distance exists between intentions and reality. One of the problems in this field is the fact that economic policies and discourses are often hardly connected to the social ones. For that reason, social experts are pledging for an integrated approach to the economic and social dimension (Mkandawire and Rodriguez 2000, Deacon *et al.* 2003, Mkandawire 2005).

5   Finally, globalization can be perceived as the emergence of a global awareness or consciousness or even identity, respecting diversity but uniting people by this shared feeling and identity (Ahmadi 2003).

Facing new realities

Globalization affects nation states and local practice to a great extent. Let us now look for a short moment at some significant issues to clarify the need for international dialogue and co-operation among social workers. Since 9/11 terrorism is believed to be one of the negative sides of a globalizing world. Cultures, identities, ethnicities, religions and economic interests are becoming more and more intermingled and by that the risk of conflicts spreading over the whole globe is increasing. Local conflicts can become global and vice versa. The penetration of Western interests and values in the heart of the Arab world created a deep rooted aversion against the dominating and infiltrating Western world. September the eleventh 2001 marked a new era in which threads from outside become threads from inside. This newly felt thread has a great impact on social policy and social work itself. Safety and security are priorities on the social agenda and social workers are assumed to co-operate in fighting against terrorism, in awareness of risks and being alert to radicalization. Another global 'evil' in this respect is the increasing trafficking of women and children exploited for sex or illegal adoption. Mobilization of people is not always about improving life conditions and creating more flexible labour markets. It implies as well new forms of slavery, illegal jobs, exploitation, and harming the integrity of the body and the mind of many vulnerable people. To what extent are social workers capable of fighting against those dark sides of mobilization and migration? What are the effects of the growing drugs, sex and trafficking industries on our cities and communities and may we expect social workers to mitigate and to prevent those interruptions in vulnerable neighbourhoods? Globalization is also connected to greater risks of environmental disasters, because of the increasing capacity of the human race to construct new risks through modern technologies, and because of the destruction of natural resources on earth (Beck 1986). Environmental disaster relief by social workers is a hot issue, in particular in the South (tsunamis, regional conflicts in Africa and Asia). Diseases, like HIV/Aids, with millions of victims, are another terrifying example of globalization. Modern mobility creates new risks in the health sector as well and again we should discuss its effects on social work practice.

The risks and opportunities in globalization are not equally met in the North and South and by the rich and the poor. It creates new tensions and greater divisions between different regions in the world and the rich and poor in all countries. It is recognizable in social work discourse as well. In the North, social work is becoming a more professionalized and recognized profession, focusing on individual responsibility and autonomy, on empowerment and activation, on change and challenge, in implementing activating welfare policies. Social workers from the South are emphasizing social justice, harmony, meaningfulness, respect, dignity and the importance of faith and religion as basics for social work (Canda 1998, Erasmus 2000, Ahmadi 2003, Zapf 2005). Other representatives of the South are stressing the political dimensions of social work: to fight against poverty, to fight capitalism, to fight the greedy society (Ife and Fiske 2006). Globalization as living in a shared world desires shared values, shared economic *and* social objectives, respecting diversity and differences. Social workers are relevant actors in implementing social objectives and social justice.

Regionalization

Globalization is affecting nation states, because they are losing control over certain economic and social politics. Multinationals and global agencies (the World Bank and IMF) are becoming more powerful, and economically the open market asks for non-intervention policies of nation states. At the same time, nation states are creating shared regional structures (EU, ASEAN) to be able to hold their strong economic position in the world. By far, the EU is the strongest and most integrated regional co-operation between independent states. As well as the EU, there is the Council of Europe, overarching all European states, not aiming however at integration.

The European Union

Aims

The European Union is basically an economic and political partnership between 27 democratic independent European states, aiming at peace, prosperity and freedom and representing nearly 500 million citizens (EU 2009). The EU focuses mainly on economic policies, creating a common market with open borders for capital, goods, services and citizens. A second common interest is foreign and security policy, aiming at Europe as a main player in international and military affairs. The third domain is fighting criminality and terrorism. An important aspect of the EU is its values, based on a number of international declarations and agreements on human, civil and social rights. Social policy, as such, is according to the subsidiary principle left to the states but since the Lisbon Declaration (2000) with its well known strategic message 'to become the most competitive and dynamic knowledge-based economy in the world capable of sustainable economic growth with more and better jobs and greater social cohesion' (Lisbon 2000) the EU accepts its overarching task to foster social cohesion by adding it to its overall ambition. In the Treaty of Lisbon 2007 a new EU foundation was created and the social cohesion and social policy notion has been clarified and expanded, as expressed in Articles 2 and 3:

Article 2

The Union is founded on the values of respect for human dignity, freedom, democracy, equality, the rule of law and respect for human rights, including the rights of persons belonging to minorities. These values are common to the Member States in a society in which pluralism, non-discrimination, tolerance, justice, solidarity and equality between women and men prevail.

Article 3

1 The Union's aim is to promote peace, its values and the well-being of its peoples.
2 The Union shall offer its citizens an area of freedom, security and justice without internal frontiers, in which the free movement of persons is ensured in conjunction with appropriate measures with respect to external border controls, asylum, immigration and the prevention and combating of crime.
3 The Union shall establish an internal market. It shall work for the sustainable development of Europe based on balanced economic growth and price stability, a highly competitive social market economy, aiming at full employment and social progress, and a high level of protection and improvement of the quality of the environment. It shall promote scientific and technological advance. It shall combat social exclusion and discrimination, and shall promote social justice and protection, equality between women and men, solidarity between generations and protection of the rights of the child. It shall promote economic, social and territorial cohesion, and solidarity among Member States. It shall respect its rich cultural and linguistic diversity, and shall ensure that Europe's cultural heritage is safeguarded and enhanced.
4 The Union shall establish an economic and monetary union whose currency is the euro.
5 In its relations with the wider world, the Union shall uphold and promote its values and interests and contribute to the protection of its citizens. It shall contribute to peace, security, the sustainable development of the Earth, solidarity and mutual respect among peoples, free and fair trade, eradication of poverty and the protection of human rights, in particular the rights of the child, as well as to the strict observance and the development of international law, including respect for the principles of the United Nations Charter.
     . . .

(Treaty on the European Union 2008)

Social policy, therefore, is unmistakably a fundamental part in the EU mission, as most explicitly expressed in Article 3.3: 'It shall combat social exclusion and discrimination, and shall promote social justice and protection, equality between women and men, solidarity between generations and protection of the rights of the child.' Besides those explicit principles and overall strategy in EU social policy, economic policies affect highly the social domain, for example, in the field of international mobility of people and services and in the privatization strategies, including services of general interest (EC 2004b). The European Court of Justice has a special influence in interpreting European laws and regulations and in conflicting regulations from different states, and has been most important in the fields of employment rights, anti-discrimination and the transferability of social security rights (Giddens 2007).

History

Europe as an identity arose in the eighteenth century in the efforts to distinguish Europe from Asia. The Turks were regarded as strangers, even after staying in Europe for over 300 years, according to Johann Gottfried Herder (Herz and Jetzlsperger 2008). At the Congress of Utrecht in 1712 the British Foreign Secretary Lord Bolingbroke spoke of the constitution of Europe and its common cause (Dunne 2008). During and after Napoleon, different European politicians, scientists and artists pledged for a European alternative for a politically fragmented Europe or a Europe conquered by Napoleon. The German Empire in 1914 and Adolf Hitler in 1939 tried, in their turn, to get power over Europe but failed as well. After the Second World War the need for a united Europe was felt as urgent to prevent a new European disastrous war. The 'Iron Curtain' and the disintegration of the Soviet superpower created a new urgency for a strong (West) Europe, based on the uniting power of Christianity, as it was expressed in this period (Herz and Jetzlsperger 2008). In 1948 Winston Churchill called for a United States of Europe at Zürich University (Council of Europe 2009b). In this light, the foundation of the European Coal and Steel Community (1951) was considered as a forerunner of a European federation of independent states, according to the Declaration of 9 May 1950 from Robert Schuman, the French Minister of Foreign Affairs in those days. France, Germany, Italy, the Netherlands, Belgium and Luxembourg were the founding members of ECSC. In 1957 the ECSC merged with two other co-operating bodies of the six countries and established the European Economic Community. Sixteen years later the UK, Ireland and Denmark joined the EEC and in 1981 Greece joined followed by Spain and Portugal in 1986. The fall of the Iron Curtain in 1989 marked a new era in Europe. The 'big enemy' to defend against disappeared and new nationalism arose in many European countries, in particular in the East and South East of Europe. On 1 November 1993 the European Union came into life, according to the Maastricht Treaty, integrating the single market represented by the EEC, the Common Foreign and Security Policy, and Justice and Home Affairs, the three 'pillars'. From a mere economic oriented ECSC evolved the EU as a partnership on economic, justice, foreign policy, security and governance issues. The open border politics (Schengen) and monetary union became part of the EU, albeit in different configurations. In 1995 Austria, Finland and Sweden joined and in 2004 ten new countries entered the EU, most of them East European States – Poland, Hungary, the Czech Republic, Slovakia, Slovenia, Estonia, Latvia and Lithuania – and the Mediterranean islands Cyprus and Malta. In 2007 Rumania and Bulgaria became members. New countries are expected to join in the coming years, starting with Croatia, Turkey and the former Yugoslav republic of Macedonia. More Balkan states will follow, and Ukraine, Morocco and Israel are looking for more involvement with the European Union. In October 2004 the 25 members of the EU signed the European Charter in Rome. The European Constitution then came into life. However, only six months later Dutch and French voters voted against it and the EU withdrew the Charter. In December 2007 the Lisbon Treaty to reform the European Union was accepted by all 27 members. This treaty was based on most central ideas of the European Charter, leaving out the symbols (flag, anthem, etc.) and the constitutional basis. In 2008 the Irish voters voted against the Lisbon Treaty but the other states decided to accept. In 2009 the Lisbon Treaty should be implemented in the EU.

Structure and governance

The EU has three main governing institutions. The European Council leads debates on conflicts, common interests and long term strategies for the EU and initiates and discusses new legislation. The European Council represents the overall leadership and consists of the heads of states (presidents) or governments (prime ministers), often accompanied by their ministers of foreign affairs. Each half year, another head of state presides over the European Council. After the implementation of the Lisbon Treaty, the European Council will get its own president for two-and-a-half-year periods, elected and appointed by the European Council. The President of the European Commission (see below) is a member of the Council as well. Besides the overarching European Council, different (sub)councils, representing the ministers of specific sectors, such as agriculture, social affairs and finance, are developing policies and legislation in those areas. Since 1979 the European Parliament has been directly elected by the EU citizens and members grouped into a number of political parties. The European Parliament is a 'co-decisive' body in legislation in certain areas together with the European Council. Gradually, the Parliament will cover more areas and perhaps obtain more decisive and controlling power. The European Commission is the executive body for preparing and implementing political strategies and decisions and steers the different directorates (ministries) by 27 commissioners, one from each member state. From 2014 onwards, the number of commissioners will be reduced to two-thirds of the members according to a rotation system. The judicial branch of the EU is mainly represented by the European Court of Justice. This court interprets and applies the treaties, laws and regulations of the EU. European laws are considered to overrule the national ones and European law is implemented directly, creating a kind of constitutional basis in the EU. The EU is based on a number of treaties, regulations and directives. Important issues are mostly prepared in green and white books to promote debates within the EU.

Some debates on the European Union

Governance and structures: the EU is unique in the world, because, on the one hand, it goes beyond regional co-operation between states and, on the other hand, it is different from a state, lacking enforcing powers, such as the police and armed forces. The balance between the EU Parliament, Council and Commission is rather complicated and asks for continuing discussions and adjustments. The dominating idea is to give gradually more power to the European Parliament but the heads of states and governments, representing independent countries, are alert on not giving too much autonomy away. Another sensitive matter is the EU bureaucracy as perceived by many observers, politicians and media in all member states. The European Commission with its directorates and directives is perceived to be regulating and thus hampers leadership. A special issue is the number of 27 commissioners to lead the directorates and the European Council. It feels like an overdone steering and fragmented leadership, due to the fact that all countries are eager 'to have their own commissioner'. A special and highly important issue is 'deficit democracy', because in a number of cases the European Council has the power to make decisions not controlled by the European Parliament nor by the national parliaments (Herz and Jetzlsperger 2008). The other democratic deficit is the lack of trust by many European citizens. European citizens are somewhat mistrusting of the European Union for its 'distance', bureaucracy, the increasing mobility of people and overruling the power of the nation state.

Civil society: the EU is mainly seen as co-operation between states and regulated by the European Parliament, Council and the Committee and its directorates. However, sovereign states are no longer exclusive members of international society (Dunne 2008) and democracy is not a system of voting and elections alone. The participative society implies that citizens are influencing and implementing policies in different structures, roles and positions. Within the EU a process of deliberations, consultations and co-operation exists between a whole array of civil society organizations. In the social field, the Platform of European Social NGOs brings together a great number of European social civil society organizations. The Platform promotes social justice and a participative society and represents the 'civil dialogue' in the social domain within the European Union. Important issues in the Social Platform are fundamental (social) rights, the debate on the privatization of social services, anti-discrimination, integration of migrants, sustainable development and the future of Europe. Apart from the civil dialogue, a social dialogue brings the social partners – employers and trade unions – together. The social dialogue focuses more or less on the same issues as the civil dialogue but emphasizes in particular issues about the labour market and working conditions in the EU.

About the EU identity

For Churchill, Schuman and many other former European-minded statesmen, Europe should develop gradually into a United States of Europe. According to the French politician Jean Monnet, the EU is not based on a blueprint but on a process of continuing deepening and widening (Herz and Jetzlsperger 2008). For other statesmen, such as Charles de Gaulle and Margeret Thatcher, Europe should be no more than a 'Europe des patries', a Europe of fully independent states, co-operating in certain fields for their own interests. Another debate is on the identity of the European citizen. In 1992 the European Union Citizenship was introduced in the Treaty of Maastricht. The central question here is whether a supranational EU citizenship is needed and to what extent. The EU territory creates an open space for moving around and asks for a set of laws, regulations, agreements and mutual adjustments between the member states. By that, all national citizens are overarched by a 'federal citizenship', guaranteeing rights and duties regarding the EU. EU citizenship is most notably present in the European Community Treaty (Maastricht), stating:

Article 8

1 Citizenship of the Union is hereby established. Every person holding the nationality of a Member State shall be a citizen of the Union.
2 Citizens of the Union shall enjoy the rights conferred by this Treaty and shall be subject to the duties imposed thereby.

Article 8a

1 Every citizen of the Union shall have the right to move and reside freely within the territory of the Member States, subject to the limitations and conditions laid down in this Treaty and by the measures adopted to give it effect . . .

Article 8b

1 Every citizen of the Union residing in a Member State of which he is not a national shall have the right to vote and to stand as a candidate at municipal elections in the Member State in which he resides, under the same conditions as nationals of that State. . . .
2 Without prejudice to Article 138(3) and to the provisions adopted for its implementation, every citizen of the Union residing in a Member State of which he is not a national shall have the right to vote and to stand as a candidate in elections to the European Parliament in the Member State in which he resides, under the same conditions as nationals of that State.

(Maastricht Treaty 1972)

In the Treaty on European Union (2008) EU citizenship is ratified again in article 9:

> In all its activities, the Union shall observe the principle of the equality of its citizens, who shall receive equal attention from its institutions, bodies, offices and agencies. Every national of a Member State shall be a citizen of the Union. Citizenship of the Union shall be additional to national citizenship and shall not replace it.

Each citizen of an EU member state is automatically an EU citizen. After accepting this (formal) citizenship, new debates arose about the social character of citizenship (Comité des Sages 1996, Dunne 2008), trying to deepen and broaden the concept of citizenship into a leading (social) concept based on social rights and social responsibility, as will be discussed in the next chapters.

About economic, environmental and social problems

Much debate among members and in EU institutions is on a whole range of economic, agricultural, environmental and social problems. A rather dominating debate is on the consequences of free movement of goods, services, capital and in particular people. International mobility is often felt as endangering national identities and creating new tensions by increasing diversity. The economic targets based on a fully open competitive European internal market are sometimes conflicting with more social issues such as cohesion, solidarity and protection of the most vulnerable people. Similar tensions are to be found between economic and environmental ambitions. The current Social Agenda focuses on two themes: full employment, and equal opportunities for all and integration. Intergenerational solidarity and strengthening trust in the EU are other topical issues within the Social Agenda. Social policy is recognized as strengthening EU economic growth and as a shared value-based EU identity.

The Council of Europe

Aims

The Council of Europe, encompassing nearly all European States (47), is older and different from the European Union. Whereas the EU was mainly based on economic co-operation, the Council of Europe was and is mainly aiming at achieving a greater understanding between its members. It is not about creating a federation of states or a comparable supranational agency or identity but a process of promoting co-operation and creating a European awareness. According to the Warsaw Summit (2005) its next objectives are defined:

1   to protect human rights, pluralist democracy and the rule of law;
2   to promote awareness and encourage the development of Europe's cultural identity and diversity;

3   to find common solutions to the challenges facing European society: such as discrimination against minorities, xenophobia, intolerance, bioethics and cloning, terrorism, trafficking in human beings, organized crime and corruption, cybercrime, violence against children;
4   To consolidate democratic stability in Europe by backing political, legislative and constitutional reform.

(Council of Europe 2009a)

History

The Council of Europe was established by the Treaty of London in 1949, from similar considerations as described in the history of the European Union. An important event – setting the tone of the Council of Europe for decades – was the Council's Convention for the Protection of Human Rights and Fundamental Freedoms. It was the first international legal instrument safeguarding human rights. In 1954 the European Cultural Convention followed, creating a framework for education, culture, youth and sport, as important areas in the Council's policies. In 1959 the European Court of Human Rights was established to ensure observance of the obligations under the European Convention of Human Rights. This Court created opportunities for citizens to claim their rights and to fight their authorities if needed. In 1990 Hungary was the first former Soviet bloc state to enter the Council of Europe. Three years later a summit of heads of state and government in Vienna adopted a declaration confirming its pan-European vocation and setting new political priorities in protecting national minorities and combating all forms of racism, xenophobia and intolerance. In 1994 the Council brought into life the Congress of Local and Regional Authorities of Europe (CLRAE) representing municipalities and regions (Länder, provinces) all over Europe. The continuing enlargement of the European Union is creating a greater overlap between the EU and the Council of Europe but the pan-European character of the Council discriminates it from the EU. In 1996 the Russian Federation became a member of the Council of Europe.

Structure and governance

The Council of Europe's structure is less complex and bureaucratic than the European Union's. Its main component parts are:

- the Committee of Ministers, the decision-making body, composed of the 47 foreign ministers or their Strasbourg-based deputies (ambassadors/permanent representatives);
- the Parliamentary Assembly for European co-operation, grouping 636 members (318 representatives and 318 substitutes) from the 47 national parliaments;
- the Congress of Local and Regional Authorities, composed of a Chamber of Local Authorities and a Chamber of Regions;
- the 1,800-strong secretariat recruited from member states, headed by a Secretary General, elected by the Parliamentary Assembly.

(Council of Europe 2009a)

The Bologna Declaration

In 1998 the Ministers of Education from France, Italy, the UK and Germany signed the so-called Sorbonne Joint Declaration stating:

> The European process has very recently moved some extremely important steps ahead. Relevant as they are, they should not make one forget that Europe is not only that of the Euro, of the banks and the economy: it must be a Europe of knowledge as well. We must strengthen and build upon the intellectual, cultural, social and technical dimensions of our continent. These have to a large extent been shaped by its universities, which continue to play a pivotal role for their development.
>
> (Sorbonne Declaration 1998)

Only one year later the Bologna Declaration was signed by 29 Ministers of Education, basically fully in line with the Sorbonne statement. The ministers stress the importance of a 'Europe of knowledge' and education. The Declaration sets a number of objectives:

- Adoption of a system of easily readable and comparable degrees, in order to promote European Citizens' employability.
- Adoption of a system essentially based on two main cycles, undergraduate (Bachelors) and graduate (Masters). The first cycle lasts for a minimum of three years.
- Establishment of a system of credits – such as the ECTS or EC system.
- Promotion of mobility for students and teachers.
- Promotion of co-operation in quality assurance (e.g. accreditation).
- Promotion of the necessary European dimensions in curriculum development, training and research.

> (Bologna Declaration 1999)

Its impact on the higher education system is remarkable, in particular in re-positioning the so-called 'Hochschule'. In most European countries the former 'Hochschule' was developing into a university of applied sciences, starting Masters courses and research centres. In different countries it endorses further integration of the 'old' and the 'new' universities. The most important consequence is the free movement of students all over Europe based on a mutual accepted system of Bachelors, Masters and credit systems.

Discussion and assignments

Discussion

- Do you have any experience of international social work in its meaning of working, or studying, across borders? If so, talk about it a little.

- Discuss the opportunities and risks of globalization.
- Do you agree with the main issues of the Bologna Declaration? Should social work education in different countries meet similar criteria and profiles?
- At US universities international social work is obligatory for Masters students. Is that a good idea? Why or why not?
- Can you give examples of EU influences on social policy and social work in your country?
- Do we need a social Europe based on shared values and laid down in a European Constitution? Why or why not?

Assignment 1

Each EU state has to regularly draft National Action Plans. Each country should have a NAP on social inclusion. Select a National Action Plan, read it, and mention the priorities on inclusion, long term care and pensions (http://ec.europa.eu/employment_social/spsi/strategy_reports_en.htm).

Assignment 2

You can find most European social NGOs on the website of the Platform of European Social NGOs (http://www.socialplatform.org/). Choose one of the members and present in two or three PowerPoint slides the essentials (aim, membership, history). You will not be able to find on the social platform website professional social associations and associations of faculties of social work and social pedagogy. You can find them on the ENSACT website (www.ensact.eu).

2 From welfare to workfare

The great transformation

Introduction

This chapter is about the significant changes in modern welfare and transition states. Those changes reflect the transformation from welfare to workfare or from Soviet bloc state to independent state. Privatization, the strengthening of civil society and localization are the three most important strategies. We shall deal with them extensively, looking at the main features and discussing their impact on national social policy and social work. Another change to take into consideration is the drastically increasing mobility and its impact on the composition of populations. Reflecting on the transformation process we can interpret it as a shift from mainly macro-economic social strategies to more socio-cultural strategies.[1]

From welfare to workfare

After the Enlightenment and the French Revolution philosophers or early sociologists wondered how integrative power could keep society together. Society (pre-French Revolution) was based on the aristocracy, the clergy, the citizens and the lower classes in a fixed system. For some social scientists the bureaucracy and the state apparatus were the powers to keep society together (Weber). Others hoped for a classless society kept together by human solidarity (Marx, Lenin). Durkheim believed in the integrative power of labour in a twofold way. First, he described society as a productive society. For him the productive state looked like a human body: each member has their own task to fulfil and together all the members are interdependent. Second, the industries are to be considered as communities (Durkheim 1986). This idea was quite popular in those days among utopians like Fourier and Owen and all kinds of productive co-operatives were established, in particular in Southern Europe. As a matter of fact, the welfare states appeared to create a rather strong integrative power by establishing nation states based on freedom, affluence, and a certain socio-economic solidarity. At the end of the twentieth century the welfare state came under pressure. Two economic recessions brought about a rethinking of the welfare state. Globalization was seen as a new phenomenon pressing states to be competitive. Decreasing public expenditure and creating work and economic activities became popular. Work,

work, work became the leading principle. The EU High Level Group advised the European Union to adjust the Lisbon Strategy by focusing fully on work and boosting the knowledge economy (EC 2004a). Instead of a priority, social cohesion and solidarity was assumed to be the outcome of the work, work, work strategy. This point of view was highly contested by the Social Platform and other European social networks and finally mitigated by the European Committee (EC 2005), but nevertheless 'work, work, work' is still the dominant strategy of the EU and its member states. The number of people on the labour market is seen as decisive for the strength and vitality of a nation.

From the 1980s the great transformation of the welfare state set in. This transformation was based on privatization, strengthening civil society and localization. State responsibilities in the social domain were transferred to the market, to citizens and to local authorities. Erroneously, this new policy has been seen as a kind of neo-liberal whim. The need for a thorough change of the welfare state has, however, been supported by nearly all the mainstream political parties in the West and adopted all over the world (Berkel and Møller 2002). This transformation can be seen as a unique impressive social innovation. However, it is not a transformation from a clear starting point A to a final destination B. It starts from a vague and unclear defined beginning without a clear blueprint as its final objective. It is indeed a transformation *process*, and presumably a continuing transformation. Social work and social professionals have to position themselves to and in this transformation process. It is not a matter of being in favour or being against the transformation process. We are in the middle of it and have to position ourselves towards and inwards of this social innovation. We can aim at redirecting the transformation, but not to stop it or to ignore it. Social professionals have to adapt to this change and should be active, creative and constructive in the discourse.

Privatization

Why privatization is popular

The privatization process of services in general interest and among them the social services has different roots. The first one is the idea, pronounced clearly by Osborne and Gaebler, to make a clear distinction between steering and rowing. In Osborne's and Gaebler's analyses the modern state was engaged too much in carrying out all kinds of rowing activities (Osborne and Gaebler 1992). In their view the state should stick to steering, giving direction and creating room for an active and alert market of profit and not-for-profit actors. Their book had a great impact on modern public managers and all over the world the nation state debate was about the role of the state and the need to get rid of all kinds of redundant tasks, services and activities provided by the state. A second argument for privatization has been put forward by international agencies as the World Trade Organization, the World Bank and the European Union. Those international bodies are urging states to be more competitive in the market and to decrease public expenditure. An important mean to that is to privatize the services of general interest. It is killing two birds with one stone. On the one hand, by privatizing services, public expenditure is decreasing remarkably and on the other hand the productive sector increases. In the European Union social services together are the second largest branch and one of the fastest growing as well. For that reason privatizing social services is highly attractive. Moreover, it should foster cost effectiveness, quality and choice. This issue of privatizing social services has been discussed vehemently in the EU during recent years (EC 2006a). The outcome of the debate is a mixed one. On the EU level privatizing social services is optional. The European Parliament rejected a formal move in this direction. The 'Bolkestein directives' (EC 2006b) were not accepted but privatization of social services is still recommended to member states and as a matter of fact is being implemented in many EU countries. The third reason is found in the idea of the overprotective state. In the period of the rising welfare state many citizens were poor and under-educated. For that reason a social protection system was developed to share risks collectively. The social protection system was a risk-sharing system in the field of pensions, children, unemployment, housing, illness and disabilities. To a great extent, access for all to education, housing, labour, health and social services has been achieved. In the postmodern state with a well educated population this collective protective system is considered outdated. It is even said to make people dependent on the protection system and its services (Marsland 1996). In the workfare state with its emphasis on activation and individual responsibility for working and living conditions a more individualized risk-taking and risk-sharing system should be more adequate (EC 1999). Most welfare states are indeed shifting certain risks from the collective sector to the privatized one.

The impact on social work

Privatization of social services is going on in a great number of EU states. In those countries the provision of social services is open to profit and not-for-profit companies and under international EU rules about tendering. There are two dominant strategies to privatizing care and welfare services. The first one is the client linked budget or personal care budget. According to Dutch research two-thirds of the clients are paying relatives, friends or neighbours for providing care for them. Ninety-five per cent of the 70,000 clients (10 per cent of all clients, 5 per cent of the overall budget) are very satisfied with this personal budget system (Velzel 2002, Ramakers and Wijngaart 2005). They like the freedom of choice and being the one to take the decisions and to employ carers or care services. The discussion is mainly on four aspects. First, freedom of choice: is it acceptable to pay for horse riding lessons or a holiday from the personal care budget? Second, how does this budget system affect informal care and the relationships with relatives and friends paid for their caring? It is to argue that personal care budgets affect the quality of the relationships in a negative way, changing informal carers (relatives or friends) into paid care workers, being 'servants' of their own relative. In *Understanding care and its future direction* some indications are found about the problem that users, in particular those with learning difficulties and some groups of mental health patients, are sometimes really bad clients, treating care workers badly (Hansen and Jensen 2004). A final problem to mention in this budgeting system is accountability, supervision and the risk of an open-ended financing system. It affects at the same time new bureaucratic regulations, hindering users and expanding controlling mechanisms. Nevertheless, the ideology of freedom of choice and independence is paramount and many users like to have a personal budget instead of a service in kind.

The second strategy for privatizing is to open a market for tendering. In most European countries, like Scandinavia, Southern European and East European countries, care services are mostly publicly organized and the shift to the open market is starting with contracting profit care providers on a small scale and by outsourcing some of the public services. In European countries, like the UK, Ireland and the Netherlands, public authorities and insurance agencies are supposed 'to purchase' social care services in an open market. The transfer is easier because those countries already had a system of independent care providers, mostly not-for-profit care institutions. Those NGOs were in general focused on a specific field of care (the disabled, the elderly, mental health, youth care, etc.) and in a specific region. They used to be financed according to fixed agreements with regional care agencies or the ministry. The system is, however, drastically changing into an open market system for not-for-profit and profit organizations alike. Permanent subvention agreements and closed markets for small groups of providers are no longer allowed. The shift into this more market oriented system will change accountability as well. Services were used to a kind of 'all in budget' related to the number of clients and the characteristics of the service. This system is changing into a budget system based on services with a fixed price. A provider has the opportunity to tender for provision of one, two or a whole range of 'products'. The institutions are no long bound to a certain target group in a certain territory. They are free to offer their products or services throughout the country and across the borders (Wistow 1996).

Privatization is already affecting the market of service providers. There is a growing market of freelancers who offer their care, act as consultants or provide other welfare services to clients or consumers (Evans and Cerny 2003). Second, an increasing market of small businesses, quite often family owned firms, are coming up with child care and care for the elderly, disabled and mental health patients, like farmers providing 24-hour care, changing their farms into guest houses for old or disabled people (Ewijk *et al.* 2002). Third, the social care institutions are opening their services to all kinds of target groups and providing them nationally or even internationally (Holden 2005). Mergers between welfare and care providers, health and care providers or social housing and care providers are becoming popular.

It is too soon to oversee fully the impact of this shift. Let us sum up the arguments for and against:

> Privatization reduces public costs but probably increases the overall budget spent on social services.

Presumably, market strategies are leading to a growing market in social welfare. People are seduced to buy social services. In the Western welfare states a market for luxury social services is developing, in particular due to wealthy elderly people and rich families who can afford private child care, luxury elderly care and mental health treatments.

Privatizing leads to more innovation and dynamics. New product–market combinations are to be expected.

Presumably privatization brings forward more choice, more effectiveness and more quality.

There are strong indications that a growing number of people have been fully excluded from services because they are not registered or not paying their fees. Under modern regimes you are excluded from social rights if you do not meet the obligations.

Privatizing strategies appeal less to volunteers and informal carers. They endanger civil society and the commitment of unpaid care workers.

More sophisticated is to reflect on the impact on the attitude and morality. It is a process of economizing the social sector or as Bob Deacon said, 'Health for all becomes health markets for all' (Deacon 2000). The effects of economizing the social sector are hardly known and hardly investigated.

Privatizing neglects and changes the character of the social domain itself. Social cohesion and social justice are in this shift interpreted as self-interest or as former Prime Minister Thatcher, talking to *Women's Own* magazine in 1987 said, 'there is no such thing as society'.

Civil society

Why civil society is popular

Civil society is often seen as the world of non-governmental organizations. There are different kind of NGOs: advocating NGOs (Amnesty International), NGOs based on common interest (scouting, sport clubs), NGOs providing volunteering services (Red Cross) and NGOs providing professional services (care providers). Sometimes the last category (the quasi NGOs or 'quangos') are not regarded as civil society but as semi-public sector. In other discourses civil society has been identified with all non-public actors, including the private market actors. We define civil society 'as representing all citizens' activities outside the public sector and market who work for the sake of the common good and common interests' (Naidoo 2003). It includes therefore among others informal care activities, informal social actions and social services provided by NGOs. In particular Putnam has emphasized the importance of a strong civil society. In his Italian research project and book *Making democracy work: civic traditions in modern Italy* he argues that regions with a lively participative civil society are much better at achieving economic and social respect. In his study he found strong arguments for the importance of a long and strong tradition in civil society as the main predictor of economic and social success (Putnam 1993). In a later study he found comparable outcomes about the achievements of American states and the involvement of civil society (Putnam 2000). It seems nowadays rather undisputed to empower civil society. It is up to the citizens to care for each other, to promote safety in neighbourhoods, to take responsibilities for leisure and to solve social tensions and social problems in their own communities (Bahmüller 2002). A second argument to strengthen civil society is from so-called communitarians who are critical about welfare regimes and welfare professionals taking over caring and social tasks belonging essentially to the community (Etzioni 2001). More neo-liberal oriented experts emphasize that social arrangements and social services are making people dependent on them instead of activating them (Marsland 1996, Zuckerman 2000). A third argument comes from community care innovation. It is forecasted and feared that in the next decades we will have a lack of hands to care because of demographic reasons (ageing, more chronically ill people), mobi-lization (distance between relatives), two-income families and changes on the labour market (lack of workers) (Cameron and Moss 2007). For that, we need the close co-operation and activation of citizens, communities and the market. If communities are falling apart, care will be at risk. Finally, we should be aware of the pressure of economizing politics. In particular, care and welfare are under discussion because the labour productivity per capita cannot increase to the same extent by technological innovation as is the case in many other sectors. The reason is that care and welfare are mainly based on face-to-face contacts and interventions. Care as service will become relatively more and more expensive.

There is a particular issue about the different roles of citizens in taking responsibilities for social services. First, citizens are supposed to care for each other, referring to informal care. Second, citizens are asked to volunteer for all kinds of activities (sports, scouting, child care, Red Cross, Amnesty International, community centres, etc.). Third, citizens are required to take steering responsi-bilities in the public sector as well as in the NGO sector, for example, being a school governor and being a member of a care supervisory board, an advisory board, and the board of a charity fund.

Active citizenship

A dominant concept in the transformation process is active or modern citizenship (Marshall and Bottomore 1992, Bauböck and Rundell 1998; Dahl 1998, Giddens 1998, Hoskins and Jeninghaus 2006). Active citizenship can be seen as a common ground for a value-shared framework for social and democratic politics. Active citizenship implies three principles:

1   The principle of self-responsibility or self-reliance. This principle refers to the idea that people should take care of their own living and working conditions and are held fully responsible for their own behaviour. They have to fulfil their duties and to behave as responsible citizens (Lorenz 2007). It is not a plea for unbridled individualism but for a conditional individualism,

based on human values such as dignity, decency and responsibility. However, this principle of self-responsibility assumes that people have resources to meet this self-responsibility. For that reason, this first principle is fully inter-dependent with the two other principles.

2   The principle of human and social rights. In a number of declarations and conventions, human and social rights are endorsed by nearly all states in the world. The social rights refer mainly to the right of access to education, labour, housing, health and a healthy environment and social protection. The activating state still endorses the rights but conditionally. The most important condition is that individuals have to meet a number of obligations. If they do not, they lose their rights. If they do not pay their health insurance contribution or rent, they lose access to health or (social) housing. The often-neglected obligation is the responsibility of local authorities to provide sufficient services and to guarantee easy access to them (Berkel *et al.* 2002). To get access the systems should be on hand (provision), have information available and be easy to access (payable, understandable, reachable).

3   The principle of social responsibility. Social responsibility refers to responsi-bility for the community, for the people around you, for caring and supporting, for social justice (Knijn and Kremer 1997, Lorenz 2006). In the Western welfare state, it is maybe the least developed principle. In the last two centuries, Western societies were very strong in liberty and equality. The eras of emancipation and progress were mainly related to this thriving power of autonomy and equal opportunities. The forgotten issue was the 'fraternity', the commitment to the community, the social dimension in life. It is now back on the European agenda by promoting social cohesion. It is actually the catchword for modern social policy and brought in by new immigrants as basic value (Ewijk 2009, pp. 8–9).

Social responsibility on different levels

Let us be a little more precise on social responsibility. The concept, together with social cohesion, is currently very popular but unclear at the same time. Sometimes social cohesion, as is the case in many EU documents, embraces mainly macro-economic social principles, like a certain share risking, a certain redistribution of income and creating a safety net. Mostly, social cohesion is in particular related to relationships between people, to connecting and bridging, and to strengthening communities. Cohesion expresses the longing for a more safe, welcoming and trusted society and community. It is interesting that those 'soft' values are becom-ing part of European, national, and local policies in particular. Social cohesion as a concept is closely linked to social responsibility. Social responsibility is the way citizens take care of each other, their communities and their social and physical environment. Social responsibility can be considered from different perspectives. A first approach to social responsibility is to ask for decent behaviour, a certain respect for each other, and to be polite. Projects about neighbourhood etiquette belong to this approach. In this approach, human relationships are dealt with as a set of codes to observe. People in society are like cars, needing a number of rules to keep it convenient for everybody. A second approach, quite close to the first, is about appealing to the *moral sense* of people. This focuses on respecting common values and observing the law. Modern leadership demonstrates a great confidence in this appeal on the moral sense (Schierup 2003, 2005). The third perspective is about *commitment*. This concerns a deeper layer in human existence. We should educate people in social commitment and in living together. Social responsibility is not only a matter of observing the rules and decency, it asks ultimately for social commitment and even social passion. Our modern school system is focused on formal education and 'learning to learn' ideas. It is underlined by the European Union in its pledge for boosting the knowledge economy. However, education should be on learning to learn *and* learning to live, including learning to live together. Healthy and strong environments need people who are educated, civilized and committed.

Contextual active citizenship

The risk of a normative active citizenship is that it measures all people in the same way. It expects every person to meet the criteria, to be fully self- and socially responsible. If citizenship does not take into account the differences between citizens, it is a discriminating concept. Therefore, we need to add that active citizenship is the basic principle for each citizen as far as it is in his or her capacity (Lister 2007). Let us take a clear example. People with very serious learning difficulties are not able to meet the criteria for a normative citizenship. Nevertheless, to treat them as active citizens is a very good idea. Modern ways of communicating and supervising start from the idea that all people, including people with serious learning difficulties, potentially have capacities to take responsibilities and to develop social competences. The same applies to frail elderly people and people with mental health (socio-psychological) disorders. Coping with them as people with the potential capacity to take their own responsibility is a constructive way of acting and thinking, however, within their capabilities. We should accept that a number of people need continuing support from their families and professionals to be active citizens. Active citizenship cannot be an argument to refuse people in need of professional support. On the contrary, contextual citizenship asks for support for vulnerable citizens to keep or get them back as active citizens. In this respect, we should introduce the principle of 'unequal treatment'. Unequal treatment means customized social support. It implies support that fits the context of this person and his or her network. Dependent on his or her 'problems' and dependent on the strength of the network and community, it will be assessed what kind of (professional) support is most appropriate (see also next chapter).

Another risk of normative citizenship in the current discourse is the one-sided focus to activation and participation as having a job, paid work. It overlooks other essential domains in activation and participation, like caring, volunteering and participation in politics and social actions. Societies are not only dependent on labour productivity but also on social productivity.

The impact on social work

The Dutch case

The idea of strengthening civil society based on activating citizenship seems to be endorsed by social professionals. It is in line with the tradition of social work itself in its concepts of empowerment, participation and emancipation. Social professionals seem fully aware of the need to activate citizens (Waal 2007). Social professionals aim to support users in taking care of themselves. Many of them refer to the fact that this approach is not new but recognize the growing stress on activation as the dominant principle of social work (Ewijk 2008). Interesting in this respect is the new Dutch Social Support Act. This Act is based on the principle that each citizen has the right and opportunity to cope with his or her own living and working conditions. It includes that each citizen is entitled to mobility in his or her own community. It refers to accessible transport, accessible public spaces, accessible public provisions and services. Another aspect of the Social Support Act is the right of each citizen to meet other people, to be a member of associations, interest clubs, etc. The Social Support Act obliges each municipality to give citizens a choice between services in kind or a personal (care) budget. In the Social Support Act it is also an obligation for all municipalities to develop a participative process of policy making. This participative process should be developed in permanent dialogue with vulnerable people. In fact we can distinguish four different fundamental rights with respect to the relationship between authorities and citizens. A first right is to be informed about the services, about the regulations, about the illness or impairment, about risks, about prognosis. In the Netherlands the right to reliable, accessible information is laid down in legislation (the Medical Treatment Agreement Act). Comparable bench marking information about the quality of services and institutions is being developed and laid down in the Social Support Act as well. A second right is to be informed about one's own medical and care files. A third right has to do with complaints and the obligation for services to have transparent procedures and standards on how to deal with complaints. A fourth right is to have a say in the provision and financing of care. National and local user representatives have the right to participate in joint consultation procedures.

Critical reflections

The discussion and criticisms in respect of civil society and citizenship are mainly on the financial impact. It is often suggested that the main drive of national governments for this transformation is based on economizing strategies. It is cutting the expenses and freeing the nation state from social responsibilities. In the US it is even quite common to suggest that an inactive state on social responsibility creates a strong civil society and strong local communities (Marsland 1996). The EU policy is up to now more based on creating a strong civil society and strong communities by an inspiring, supportive European social strategy and endorsing national strategies as well (Lisbon European Council 2000). However, actually, Europe is more focused on economic growth and boosting the knowledge economy than on strengthening civil society. Professionals and other experts, from their side, are critical about the fact that civil society and citizen 'ideology' neglects the very vulnerable groups in society, such as children, the frail elderly, seriously disabled people and people with serious mental health problems. They stress the permanent need for a strong support system for those people and are afraid of overrating the social capacities of marginal people. Another aspect under discussion is the suggestion that care, social support and social intervention are equally to be taken care of by citizens or professionals. This neglects the professional competence needed for specific interventions and in complex situations. Another comment on civil society empowerment is the fear that it will affect mostly women, because they are the main providers of care and welfare. And additional to this argument, it is said that informal carers and volunteers are already heavenly engaged and it is felt as unreasonable to load them even more. Civil society policies often neglect the fact that in many areas care and social support are already mainly organized and carried out by citizens. It could be felt as overlooking and overcharging informal carers and volunteers.

Localization

Why localization is popular

The third strategy from the nation state is to shift from the national level to the regional and in particular to the local level. The dominating idea is that modern social problems are mostly contextual with a strong individualized component and a community or network component. Contextual problems need integrative approaches, bringing different sectors and services together. The user should be the focus point, not a specific service or special profession. For that reason local embedded social politics and social services are more adequate than national strategies and services. Localization of social policy and social work, bringing them closer to the citizen, is another argument. National policies are hardly influenced by locally organized citizens. The rediscovery of the local community is remarkable. As we have seen, the classic sociologists sought the integrative power of society in central administration, classless society or labour and industries as communities. It is worth analysing this move to the local community a little deeper. Many modern urban planners and investors in housing are highly aware of the economic value of a neighbourhood, a district or a city. Investments are losing their value if neighbourhoods impoverish, if there are serious conflicts or a lack of facilities. The value of a neighbourhood is not only in physical capital and economic activities; there is an important added value in the social climate. In the big cities the effect of upgrading marginal neighbourhoods is measured and compared with other neighbourhoods. Not only are states seen as more competitive. Cities and districts are competing as well. Putnam's *Bowling alone* (2000) shows that investments of citizens in taking care of the neighbourhood and to care for each other are very cost effective in preventing professional intervention.

Another reason can be found in the overwhelming evidence that modern citizens expect to live in safe and convenient surroundings. Lifestyle arguments matter maybe most in choosing where to live. The growth of popular right-wing political parties is partly to consider as reacting to neglecting the quality of the living conditions in neighbourhoods.

The impact on social work

In a number of European countries, such as Finland and Denmark, social care, youth and child care and social assistance have been local responsibilities for a long time. In many other European countries the shift has set in recently. We find a number of problems in devolution and localization (see Chapter 5). A first issue is the fact that local authorities often lack the decision-making power, the budget and the capacity to co-ordinate and implement those complex objectives. In the private market, very strong and big companies are coming up with a lot more capital and expertise than the average municipalities. Also, a number of governmental and national sectors are still fully under national control. Local authorities are expected to co-ordinate and integrate those 'powers' but lack regulative and financial power. A problem of a different order is caused by the fact that localization and contextualization are open for new inequalities. Poor municipalities and problematic neighbourhoods cannot compete with rich and resourceful municipalities. It becomes even more difficult as the overall strategy aims at empowering communities to self-development. It is asking the poor and excluded communities to compete with the much more resourceful communities. National systems of redistribution are certainly needed. However, accepting a certain inequality – mitigating a strong equality ideology – is sensible to a certain degree.

On the positive side, localization seems to foster more integrative ways of dealing with complex situations. Many local authorities and local services are creative and constructive in finding new answers to this transformation process. Localization and devolution contribute to integrative approaches and blurring borders between sectors, services and professions. It is interesting to see that in many countries integration processes are going on in different areas of social welfare. In social education, schools, youth care, leisure time services, families and family support systems and even urban planning agencies are working together to create a strong, challenging and consistent social educational context. In social care for elderly, disabled, homeless and mental patients, integration of housing, care and welfare services is going on to build strong, caring communities. Prevention, intervention, socio-cultural (for example, community art) and recreational activities are coming together to empower the community and to foster safety, vitality and cohesion (Eijken and Ewijk 2005).

Conflicting strategies

In countries which have made big steps in the triangle strategy of privatization, localization and citizenship, like the UK, Ireland and the Netherlands, local authorities are caught in two conflicting strategies. On one hand they are pressed to privatize social services, on the other they are expected to foster civil society and activating citizenship. Most municipalities are embracing the market approach and the community approach at the same time but often without a sensible coherent strategy. Social professionals feel the tensions between vertical and horizontal mechanisms and market and community mechanisms. Let us reflect a little more on this strategy.

The community strategy

The users and social professional relationships in the community approach is to characterize as a citizen–community (society) relationship. Citizens are not seen as mere consumers but as people living in a certain context. When they have serious problems or are in need of care, the community (neighbourhood, family and friends) should be taken as a starting point for support and intervention. The community and networks are essential for effective intervention and prevention (OECD 1999). In the community approach, a certain territory is seen as a kind of managerial area. It does not mean that people are not taking part in all kinds of other communities going beyond the neighbourhood territory but the neighbourhood as territory where people live is a promising way for social monitoring, social support and social interventions. Particularly, vulnerable people and children are often dependent on their own local context. Partnership between the local authorities, all kinds of providers and civil society – referring to citizens in organized volunteering settings and in informal settings where they take care of their social and physical surroundings – is the key to the community approach and this partnership is based on trust (DV 2001). To trust social workers and giving them discretional room for their professionalism is one of the basic principles. Accountability for their interventions and support is the counterbalancing principle. Professionals are supposed to work through the community, rather than on the community (Banks 2006). Social managing of a neighbourhood is based on integrated domains (zones) in social care, social education and community development, each of them managed by recognizable services and steered towards partnership. A local community can create a co-operative structure (citizens, professionals, public sector) to foster, monitor and stimulate the community in taking its responsibilities. It is about looking (eyes), listening (ears), taking the initiative (hands), collecting, enriching and disseminating knowledge (brains) and to be really involved in and committed to the community (heart).

The market strategy

The market strategy starting point is opposite to the community approach. The fundamental basis is the consumer–producer relationship. In this relationship freedom of choice, cost effectiveness and quality are the presumed outcomes (EC 2005). It requires an open market where all kinds of competing providers are offering their services to the citizens. As a matter of fact in the social and care

Table 2.1 The community market schedule

Community strategy	Market strategy
Citizen–community (society)	Consumer–producer
Integrated, contextual approach	Competing providers offering services
Territorial, community based	Not territorially oriented
Partnership of authorities, professionals and citizens	Entrepreneurship, contracts, competition
Based on trust	Based on market mechanism
Different 'zones' (care, social education, neighbourhood approach) with a managing centre directed in partnership	Imprecise market of services, sometimes coming together in service centres based on outsourcing and contracting
Creating agencies of professionals and citizens, being the 'ears, eyes, heart, hands and brains' in the community	Aiming at cost effectiveness and maximum choice

domain, certain services are 'purchased' by collective identities as local authorities or insurance companies, but this does not need to hamper marketing strategies. A market oriented service provider is aiming at entrepreneurship, innovation and developing new markets. The state and municipality regulate this market to a certain extent, for example, to create a level playing field (EC 1999). Successful enterprises are upgrading their territorial scale (from local to regional to national and global) and are quite often expanding their core business to adjacent areas. Sometimes enterprises work together in a kind of supermarket model in a neighbourhood centre but only as long as it is profitable. The market model has problems in attracting volunteers and most social professionals because the basic principle of profit making is not appealing to them. On the other hand, for more innovating and enterprising social workers it could be very attractive to expand this market orientation.

Reconciling the strategies

The thing to be done is to find a sensible mix of both strategies in a creative and effective way. To hang fully on one side is unrealistic and even not productive. There is enough room for innovating market oriented services and a basic public community infrastructure. Local communities need a simple and plain but strong basic structure based on the community approach. Those structures are managing the different 'zones', providing the basic services by generalist front line workers and should represent the eyes, ears, hands, brains and heart of the community. This basic structure should be transparent, recognizable and very accessible for all citizens, in particular for the most needy. The emphasis lies on 'to be known and knowing what is going on', on information, consultation, and reference, and on direct intervention when needed. Assessment of problems and contexts belongs to the competence of the basic structure and front line social professionals. Around, additional and next to this basic structure, we find a 'fuzzy' market of all kinds of providers and for all kinds of services in the field of care, social education and (social) cultural activities. Even specialized institutions in care, mental health and youth care can be privatized if the basic local structure is well enough organized. This implies the creation of a profit-oriented market in the domain of care and social support, attractive for more entrepreneurship-oriented professionals and all kinds of specialists and back-up offices, besides a public or semi-public basic front line infrastructure.

Integration

Why integration is discussed so much

Along with the transformation of the welfare state most European countries have been confronted with global and EU internal mobility of people. Populations are becoming mixed at an increasing pace and it is causing uneasiness in different respects. In particular the immigration of African and Asian people has been felt as problematic in the Western world. The enlargement of the European Union contributes to an acceleration of migration within the EU. About this phenomenon of integration, concepts such as multicultural and intercultural approaches are becoming popular. Before discussing the concepts it is useful to break down the massive integration discourse into a number of separate 'problems', related to and connected with integration. The different 'problems' need different strategies. However, the risk is to add up all the elements and increase the integration discourse to a kind of massive and problem-oriented debate on migration, integration and multiculturalism.

Elements

On the one hand, looking into the integration debate we often find incident-related discussions and, on the other hand, theoretical – if not ideological – debates on which perspective should be accepted by society on integration and migration. In this first section we will deal with integration as a multi-faceted area.

Smooth integration

On average about half of the migrants are migrants from neighbouring welfare or transition states and actually cause hardly any problems. In the Netherlands British people, unable and perhaps willing to speak Dutch, are highly integrated and accepted. Many people from overseas countries are doing quite well. They learn the language, adopt Western habits and values and respect their own background. They are rather successful in education and on the labour market. Maybe 80 to 90 per cent of the immigrants are easily integrated. In this respect immigrants and international mobility contributes to more flexible and dynamic societies and discussing the 'multicultural drama' (Scheffer 2007) is debatable because it refers to a minority of the ethnic minorities.

Brain drain

Looking at migration, Western Europeans are inclined to relate integration with the immigration of badly educated African and Asian immigrants. In East European countries migration is partly associated with the emigration of academics and skilled personnel. Their basic problem is that residents, in whom the state invested most, are leaving the country. It is a matter of disinvestment and losing the academic and skilled population. On the other hand, going abroad can enrich the national economy and knowledge as well, in particular if people are coming back or at least are keeping their economic and intellectual connections with the country they come from.

Parallel societies

Parallel societies refer originally to a legal and established society and an illegal but lively second society, such as the 'favella' in Rio de Janeiro. Being in New York one can notice how different (but legal) societies are living together and at the same time are highly separate from each other. The Spanish community is speaking Spanish only, having their own schools and structures but feeling themselves fully American. In Europe parallel societies are coming up and we have to position ourselves towards this development (Nowak 2006). As a matter of fact, some small parallel societies were already existing, such as the Chinese community, but confronted with new African and Asian communities the question is becoming more urgent if we are going to accept parallel societies and to what extent.

Exclusion

Exclusive mechanisms are always there in societies and there are always individuals or groups who prefer to be more or less excluded. The problem in the integration debate is the increasing number of new migrants who are willing but not able to enter the labour market or to succeed in education. On the one hand, some of the migrants are lacking the educational and social competences to integrate in society. On the other hand, Western societies are not very open for African and Asian migrants. The process of exclusion seems to harden and the number of excluded migrants grows.

Illegality

A specific aspect and a little different from parallel societies and exclusion are the illegal immigrants who lack permission to live in the country and as such are considered as non-existent in statistics and in the field of human and social rights. In the tougher modern society being tolerant of and welcoming to illegal persons is no longer acceptable. Even churches are challenged by politicians if they offer illegal immigrants shelter and food.

Hard criminal core

Criminal gangs and brutal, offensive and violent behaviour are not new in modern society. The new thing is that they are more associated with the integration problem, supported by the fact that in the figures migrant backgrounds are over-represented. In particular, groups of young African, Asian or far-East European males are felt as threatening, and contaminating the overall picture of migrants. The link between cultural and ethnic origin and the inclination to criminal and maladjusted behaviour is quickly made, but erroneously (Wacquant, 1999). It makes more sense to explain over-representation of ethnic groups in criminal statistics as a consequence of economic mechanisms, discrimination, drastic cultural change and lack of educational and modern welfare state social competences.

Religious radicalism and terrorism

Religious fanaticism and terrorism are not by definition related to each other. Since 11 September 2001 the link is easily made. The coming together of Muslim radicalism and Muslim terrorism is frightening Western societies. Integration and the risk of terrorism are associated and create a negative impact on current concepts of integration and migration. Are we hosting a hostile, potentially endangering world in European society is the probing question, put by politicians, media, scientists and many other citizens (Huntington 1997, Ayaan 2006).

The clash of civilizations

After Huntington's book suggesting a clash to come, we cannot deny a risk of hostile civilizations (1997). Here it is not only about a specific group of people threatening Western society but about a conflict between the Muslim world and the Western Christian-based world. The fear of this clash is even dominating discussions on earthly things like wearing a veil or not shaking hands.

Perspectives

After having deconstructed the integration discourse in different elements to consider separately, we will move on to the perspectives on integration as such. Integration stands for bridging between different (ethnic) groups in society and creating a level playing field. Integration is endangered if too many of the ethnic minorities are not participating or behaving in a hostile manner in our societies. Integration is even more endangered if the dominant ethnic group(s) is excluding or even explicitly discriminating against minorities. Or to put it in another way, a hostile society and an excluding national migration strategy are opposite to a positive and empowering integration strategy and are changing social workers into gatekeepers and controllers (Hayes and Humphries 2006). Discussing perspectives on immigration should consider positive and negative perspectives. Integration as such is broader than discussing ethnic groups. Nevertheless, nowadays, the focus is mainly on ethnicity in the integration debate. We shall now distinguish four main perspectives.

Discrimination

Discrimination has been a formally non-existent political perspective in many welfare states for many years. It is changing now. New right-wing political parties are openly asking for more discriminating policies regarding ethnic groups. This is not only in respect of illegal aliens or new migrants but of migrants who have already obtained full citizenship, for example, in respect of marriage, criminal behaviour and even mobility (regulations about the maximum number of migrants to live in a certain neighbourhood). Discrimination is becoming an acceptable perspective in political debates (Nimako 2002). Discrimination is often distinguished in direct and indirect discrimination. Direct discrimination means being openly discriminative to certain persons or groups of people. Indirect discrimination refers to the effects of certain policies and attitudes that exclude or hinder people.

Normalization and assimilation

Assimilation starts from the idea that all inhabitants have to meet the demands of a certain society and migrants have to adjust fully to the dominating culture, the values and ethics. It hardly leaves room for specific ethnic-related behaviour, culture and ceremonies. The emphasis is on becoming 'as us'. Normalization is quite often associated with assimilation. It is considered as a process of adjustment as well. Normalization as a concept, however, became popular in the world of people with learning disabilities in the 1960s (Bengtson *et al.* 2003). It was discussing the protection paradigm and stood for accepting disabled people as equals. The emphasis was on equal (social) rights and creating a level playing field. Disabled people should have the opportunity to participate in all aspects of society. For that reason, normalization is more than adjusting to a dominating culture. It was much more about accepting different groups in normal society and giving them full access. The negative connotation of normalization is due to the word 'normal', suggesting that there is a kind of (Western) standard of human behaviour everybody should adapt to.

Diversity, multicultural and intercultural perspectives

Throwing diversity, multicultural and intercultural perspectives together is a little unfair and not answering properly the extensive literature on those aspects. Nevertheless, there are common features and ideas. Diversity is a broader option than multiculturality, referring to all kind of diversities, not only the ethnic cultural ones (Banks and Banks 1989, Gutiérrez *et al.* 2005,). Interculturality, on the other side, stresses more the need to connect different cultures to each other. However, the main perspective in all three concepts is on respect for different cultures and regarding them as equal in human value (Erickson 1992, Taylor 1992). All three perspectives request recognition of different cultures and the right to be oneself in private life and as much as possible in public life. This approach has been contested because the right to be different suggests it is leading to the right to indifference, to accept the current situation (Bauman 2001, Lorenz 2006). Therefore, multiculturalism also needs to imply the normalization thesis as far as it is about equal access and equal rights and about promoting exchange and connection between different ethnicities (Lorenz 2006). In Giddens's words: [Multicultural policy recognizes . . .] 'the authenticity of different ways of life within a social community, and seek to promote fruitful and positive transactions between them – but within an overall, and singular, system of citizenship rights and obligations' (Giddens 2007:124).

The multi-actor perspective

The multi-actor is closely related to the former one on diversity. It fully respects different cultures and the equal value between them. The specific quality is to emphasize the need for looking at people, problems and incidents from different angles (Kortram 2004). Discussing youth problems the public and political debate is mainly on the violent behaviour of certain groups of young people. It oversees the fact that (those) young people themselves are more victims of abuse and violence by adults than the other way round. Discussing problems of youth behaviour should be multi-perspective to reflect the real situations and problems. Incidents about wearing a veil can only be solved within a specific context and should be discussed by the relevant actors, listening to each other. In many debates about integration the political representatives discuss the problem of ethnic minorities by referring to an 'us' and 'them' perspective, ignoring the fact that those 'minorities' are already an integrated part of our society and belong to 'us'.

And not only is the multi-perspective essential; to be sensitive to the fact that ethnicity is only one of the characteristics is essential as well. Each person is a mix of characteristics. Ethnicity, age, gender, physical features, intelligence and so on together create a mixed identity and dependent on the context and the person some characteristics are felt as most decisive. Stereotyping people into only one category is overemphasizing one aspect.

The impact on social work

The mixing of populations has been most keenly felt in poor areas and marginal neighbourhoods for two reasons. The first one is that exactly in those areas the changes in the population and the loss of existing integrating structures are most drastic. The second reason is that selective mechanisms within ethnic groups and among the original populations cause a quick impoverishment of those areas, because the more wealthy leave the most deprived areas. The heat of integration conflicts (illegality, hard core criminality, the clash between different ethnic identities) is particularly in those deprived areas. In this respect migration sometimes produces alarming effects in a relatively small number of certain districts or neighbourhoods. Integration as a threatening process is hardly present in the majority of municipalities and neighbourhoods. It is a specific problem in specific areas. However, in those territories it requests concentrated interventions and cohesive strategies including influencing the composition of the population in those areas. Another fact to consider is the change in politics towards refugees, nowadays called asylum seekers. Many more restrictive policies are adopted by nearly all European countries, and social workers are expected to answer to those new policies, changing their role as gatekeepers, and agents of inspection (Hayes and Humphries 2006). Apart from those specific problems in specific areas, integration should not and need not be a specific field of social work. It asks for some national strategies to prevent labelling processes and open debates about conflicting issues. And we need to facilitate the integration of new migrants. The shadow of a clash of civilizations and the fear of a rising world of religious fanaticism connected with terrorism needs an alert awareness and counterbalancing perspectives. It is definitely not a problem of two conflicting civilizations alone. Maybe the hardening is much more a common feature in both 'civilizations' than between them and, therefore, needs to be dealt with in a close partnership between the different 'civilizations'. The reality and concept of diversity is at the same time affecting social welfare and should be answered by new concepts, methods, attitudes and competences within the social services. And within the services the workforce is changing and adapting to the new mix at the same time (see Chapter 7).

From a macro socio-economic strategy to a micro socio-cultural strategy

Concluding this chapter on the European states in transformation, we shall summarize the main features and interpret them as a shift from national macro socio-economic strategies to localized, privatized and citizen oriented socio-cultural ones.

Summary

The starting question was about the integrative power of society. Characteristic of the postwar and post-communist-soviet period is the multilevel approach of cohesive strength. The levels are: global (UN), regional (EU), national, county-level and local. A certain shift from national to international and from national to local is going on. Work, the old Durkheimian concept of labour as binding in productive states and industries as communities, and the local community are maybe the most emphasized integrative powers of postmodern societies. We discussed the Western obsession with freedom and equality, neglecting brotherhood or cohesion. Three dominant shifts have been analysed: privatization, civil society and localization. Privatization includes new managerial ideas about steering and rowing, transferring public expenses in market profits and making people more independent and more risk taking. The impact of privatization is on new ways of financing, creating an open market and changing social dimensions into economic ones. Strengthening civil society comes from studies demonstrating that active civil society promotes economic results and strengthens democracy. Basically, in civil society is the modern concept of citizenship based on self-responsibility, social responsibility and social rights. Social responsibility is the modern catchword and is related to social cohesion and participation. The discussion is mainly on the risk of overcharging people and overestimating the capacities of certain groups of citizens. Localization is based on the idea that contextual approaches are needed to deal with social and care problems. Contextual approaches need integration of services. Care and case management approaches can be best organized at the local level. Another line of argument is on the competitive power of territorial areas (states, cities, neighbourhoods). An area can be seen as a territory to invest in. Localization creates steering problems in co-ordination, often lacks expertise and capacity and causes inequalities between areas. On the positive side, integrative developments are to seen in different domains, such as long term care, social education and community development. Finally we discussed the tension between privatization and strengthening civil society. The other transformation process states are in is about mobilization, migration and integration of different groups of people in society. We split up this process in different aspects, from smooth and easy integration to the threat of clashing civilizations and dealt with different perspectives on integration: discrimination, normalization, diversity and the multi-actor approach.

Is the nation state losing its social interest?

Social expenditure belongs in welfare states to the most consuming national budgets. Privatizing, handing it over to civil society and localization are taking over the social responsibility and reducing the national budgets on social protection. A certain redistribution of income, labour and social expenditure and a certain collective social risk sharing will be kept as a national responsibility but this aspect of social politics is becoming rather technical in welfare states. It asks for the regulative power of the nation state but does not appeal to social commitment and social debates. For that reason, it is feared that nation states are losing their social interest and will even be more focused on fostering economic growth and boosting the knowledge economy. It creates a lack of social leadership on the national level, leaving social and caring issues to the local authorities, civil society and the market on the one hand and EU rhetoric on the other hand.

The shift to micro socio-cultural strategies: a personal reflection

In the last two centuries, the dominant social issue was to raise the level of education, to civilize the populations and to create preventive and risk sharing socio-economic systems, like the pension system, unemployment benefits, social assistance, child benefits and health assurance. The driving and continuing conflicting basic ideologies were rooted in the concepts of freedom and equality. This brought forward the welfare state, bridging the concepts. At the beginning of the twenty-first century the 'social quest' could be moving from a dominant socio-economic approach to a much more socio-cultural one. The 'work, work, work' mantra embraces activation programmes in the domains of work, care, civil society and the public arena. Since 9/11 the Western world seems to be even more in the grip of a much more socio-cultural quest on how to keep people and societies together, how to prevent extremism, hard criminality, extreme behaviour. Opinion polls about people's concerns refer to issues such as health, relationships, violence, and problematic behaviour. Even poverty and unemployment are perceived as an individual or group-related lack of social competences (Room 1995). At the end of the 1980s the EU replaced the word 'poverty' by 'exclusion', shifting the emphasis from economic argument to social reasoning (Berkel *et al.* 2002). There is a feeling that modern individualism has surpassed its limits. The greedy individual, the offensive individual, the not-respecting individual and the identification of freedom with free riding in society are heavily criticized (Sennet 1977, Beck 1986, Giddens 1991, 1998, Marsland 1996). Political leaders call for a more committed and moral attitude. We are looking for a certain rethinking of individualism in the postmodern world. We fear a hardening of relationships and an increase in indifferent social behaviour by individual persons. The longing for a world to feel at home in is a very recognizable feeling (Bauman 2001). We need more bridging capacities between and among people. The bridging competency stands for the quality to connect between different groups, different people, and different situations.

The EU strategy of promoting wealth and knowledge push and creating a more social world by that is based on the classic social quest: education and work create a better and more cohesive world. Titmuss already analysed that this ideology was debatable, because it does not solve inequality and creates new problems (Alcock 2001). Indeed, progress in welfare creates new opportunities and often a more congenial world to live in. However, the affluent society is a difficult one to live in for other reasons. Progress in wealth and knowledge progress create new demands, basically in a more socio-cultural perspective. 'We are all, in some senses, victims and offenders, confronted as we are with the problem of the growth of knowledge in complex societies and the division of intellectual labour into smaller and smaller segments' argued Titmuss (Alcock 2001:164). An open, complex, and ever changing society and community asks for competences to be mobile, flexible, and to answer new demands in knowledge, attitude and skills. The new world is more secure in obtaining food, shelter, education, comfort, but insecure in its relationships, communities, religious and ideological systems. Many young people are missing a goal or motivating aim in their life. The number of people in prisons, in mental health institutions, in youth care is rising. Many citizens are less rooted in their life and environment. The world around is even felt as inhospitable (Lane 2000). It is said that modern or postmodern people need different identities at the same time and people need to participate in different communities and networks. The idea is that weak ties are more useful than strong ties (Putnam 2000). A successful person has a whole array of connections and contacts. A too strongly tied person, or community, is hampering full integration into society. It looks like expecting people to be flexible and creative without a firm anchor in a sustainable and supportive community, demanding the utmost of many citizens. Another phenomenon of the socio-cultural society is that feelings, experiences, behaviour and relationships are counting most. Facts become constructions, contexts become choices, and sensibility becomes sensitivity. The impact of this new era is the need for many people to be supported and helped in their paths through life and society. Social problems are socio-cultural ones, not asking for systems and systematic solutions, not asking for cure and treatment, but for personal, context-related interventions and support. However, this more socio-cultural society assumes, and let that be very clear, a macro economic system for social protection and access to education, health, work, housing and social protection. The socio-cultural society is absolutely dependent on a firm socio-economic basis. The transformation from a welfare state to a workfare state should be changed into a transformation from a welfare state based on freedom and equality (state and individual person) into an activating welfare state based on freedom, equality and cohesion (state, individual and community)

Therefore, modern social work in welfare states is moving from socio-economic and emancipative practices to more personal and contextual socio-cultural approaches, based on a socio-economic basis and on adequate social rights for all. Human growth and progress are no longer identified with the great ideologies but with living and connecting in a complex and highly diverse world. Localization, citizenship and communities, social capital, cohesion, social competences, supporting and enabling are leading concepts in our work.

Discussion and assignment

Discussion

Transformation process

Do you recognize the transformation process? Could you discuss the differences between the transformation from a welfare state to a workfare state and from a former communist state to a workfare state? Is it true that we are moving from a more socio-economic social policy to a more socio-cultural one? Do you understand and agree with the idea of the activating welfare state?

Privatization

Can you reflect on the argument on economizing the social dimension? What do you think about the impact of privatization on the social work profession? Can you reflect on the impact of privatization of social services in your own country?

Civil society

Do you know to what extent strengthening civil society and modern (activating) citizenship are important issues in your country? What are their national and/or local influences on local responsibilities and duties of its citizens? Can you reflect on your ideas about the three pillars of citizenship as introduced in this section? What do you see as the impact of civil society and citizenship on the social work profession?

Localization

Can you describe to what extent local authorities are responsible for social and care policies in your own city or village? What are the strengths and weaknesses in the localization of social policies? Discuss the market and community approach and their strong and weak points. Do you think the idea of a basic local social infrastructure and room for private companies 'around' this structure is a good idea?

Diversity

What do we think about parallel society, a growing divide between different cultures, about terrorism and religious radicalism? Are social professionals capable and willing to meet the demands of fighting against criminality by young ethnic gangs, of helping in the war against terrorism, in getting more ethnic minority people integrated into education, health, social protection, housing and labour systems? Discuss the four perspectives and your opinions on the different perspectives.

Assignment

Draft a short essay (about three pages) commenting on the five topics outlined above.

3 Citizenship and civil society discourse

Helene Jacobson Pettersson and Hans van Ewijk

Introduction

In Chapter 2 we discussed civil society as one of the driving concepts in the transformation process European countries are going through. We referred to the European political interpretation of citizenship, stressing self-responsibility for the personal living and working conditions, fighting against a presumed over-invasive welfare state making citizens dependent, and social responsibility, implying a shared responsibility of citizens in their communities and in society. This interpretation of citizenship connects to 'social citizenship', a concept brought in by Marshall. In this chapter we reflect on social citizenship, its concepts, its history, its discourse. After a short overview on citizenship and civil society in general, we will deal in particular with social citizenship, starting with Thomas Humphrey Marshalls' original triad – civil, political and social citizenship (Marshall 1950) – and Tom Bottomore's distinction between formal and substantial social citizenship (Marshall and Bottomore 1992). From there, we discuss Ruth Lister's feminist point of view and her focus on differentiated universalism and subjective citizenship (Lister 2003, 2007), and at the end we will come back to activating citizenship, its strengths and weaknesses.

Citizenship and civil society

Citizenship has a long history in Western political thinking since the classical Greek polis (Turner 1993). In the days of Socrates, Plato and Aristotle, citizenship was seen as a civic duty and deeply rooted in virtue, if needed, in sacrificing life for the sake of the polis (Keller 2003). In Roman times citizenship was perceived in its more legal position and based on universal laws (Cicero). In Greek and Roman times citizenship was a privilege for a minority, for males and by birth or class. In early Christian times all people – at least the converted – belonged to the Civitas Dei (Augustine). Citizenship as a political idea about the roles and responsibilities of people in society was not so much on the agenda in medieval times. As a matter of fact, citizenship and civil society ideas and practice survived in certain areas in Europe but came back on the agenda, starting with John Locke who distinguished state and civil society as different entities (Locke (1689) cited in Brink 1994). The discourse focused on the question of whether the state is a prerequisite for civil society or an active civil society is a prerequisite for a successful state. The divide between the state and other public domains created the idea of the trias politicas: the executive, the legislative and the judicial. Civil society – 'corps intermédiaires' – could fill the gap between those powers and the individual. In the twentieth century, three dominating perspectives developed: social liberalism, communitarians and radical democrats.

Social liberalism is characterized by Dahrendorf's quote:

> The search for a civil society, and ultimately a world civil society, is one for equal rights in a constitutional framework which domesticates power so that all can enjoy citizenship as a foundation for their life changes.
>
> (Dahrendorf 1988: 34–5)

Maybe the word 'enjoy' is misleading, because it should be read as 'realize' at the same time. Citizens are agencies of civil society within the constitutional framework enabling this civil society. Civil, political and social rights create the essentials for the civilized world. In particular the values and norms are not dictated by the authorities but developed by continuous deliberations among citizens. Dahrendorf believed in individual perspectives and pluralism, and not in a collective ideal and morality. 'The task of liberty is to work, and if needed to fight, for an increase in life chances', Dahrendorf argued (1988: 18). Dahrendorf stresses the representative democracy and was critical about the republican idea of an explicit political community (Brink 1994).

Communitarism concentrates on the relationship between citizens and community and sociability as human motivation.

> The picture [of civil society] . . . is of people associating and communicating with one another, forming and reforming groups of all sorts, not for the sake of any particular formation – family, tribe, nation, religion, commune, brotherhood or sisterhood, interest group or ideological movement – but for the sake of sociability itself. For we are by nature social, before we are political or economic beings.
>
> (Walzer (1991) cited in Brink 1994)

Sociability is the primary overall objective for society. Walzer challenges the individualistic and utilitarian tendency in modern society and starts from a pluralistic society that asks for balancing and overarching different settings.

> The citizen must be ready and able, when his time comes, to deliberate with his fellows, listen and be listened to, take responsibility for what he says and does. Ready and able: not only in States, cities, and towns but wherever power is exercised, in companies and factories, too, and in unions, faculties, and professions.
>
> (Walzer (1983) cited in Brink 1994)

Radical democracy comes from the heritage of the Frankfurt School with its strong ideas about social justice, universal values and sovereignty by the people, fighting against a society based on consumerism and mass culture. They opt for democratic control by all citizens. As Marx and Engels, Habermas and others thought, civil society was not that important, for it could be seen as a threat to a full democratic political system. Civil society was considered as representing certain issues, themes and signals from citizens but not as an integral part of the political system.

The ideological debate between the different schools died away in the last decades. Postmodern ideas and 'the end of ideologies' created a climate for more contextual and pragmatic approaches. It reopened the discourse about civil society and its role in a modern globalizing and localizing world from different angles. A first debate is on the character and definition of civil society. The recognized characteristics are 'voluntary', 'citizens' activities', 'not market and not public sector', and 'for the sake of common goods and common interests' (Naidoo 2003). However, the problem is that in practice, borders are blurring between public sector and NGOs, since many NGOs are highly dependent on financing by the public sector, and borders are blurred between civil society activities and market activities, since both are competing in the market. The civil society concept is rather complicated, leading to vehement discussion about who is and who is not representing civil society. A second debate is about the role and responsibility of civil society. Because 'voluntary work' is a dominant characteristic of NGOs, it is hard to position and to profile civil society as a fully responsible actor for creating and carrying out social policies.

We find in European countries practice close to the radical democrats – bringing back civil society to signalling and bringing forward thematic issues – for a long time a feature in the Nordic countries. In the German-speaking countries we find the practice of NGOs as professional providers of social services. In Eastern Europe civil society is less organized and fighting for recognition. In EU politics, as in most EU countries nowadays, civil society is seen as an important actor in decision-making processes and in carrying out core social tasks in society. By that, many NGOs and parts of civil society are becoming actors within the public system on the one hand, and actors competing in the market with not-for-profit firms as well. Therefore, we see two movements at the same time: strengthening civil society in the modern European context and blurring borders between civil society, market and public sector.

Perspectives on citizenship

In the comprised overview of civil society we recognize in the debates the different perspectives on citizenship:

1   Citizenship as status and privilege (Greece, Rome). For a long time citizenship was an exclusive position, reserved for a specific group. In postmodern times citizenship is felt to be more inclusive, albeit excluding people with the

'wrong' nationality or without a permit to live in a specific country, the so-called 'denizens' (Hammar 1990).

2   Legally based citizenship, often named 'classical liberal' citizenship, refers to a set of civil and political rights. Citizenship is restricted to the juridical and public domain and refers to a formal position. This was contested by Dahrendorf, as we saw.

3   Social citizenship – or the social liberal approach – (Marshall, Dahrendorf), adding to the civil and political rights the social ones, mainly related to access to the main domains of social life: education, health, housing, work and social security.

4   Virtue-based citizenship, often named 'republican' and 'neo-republican'. The emphasis is on citizens as active agencies who elect and control the government and local authorities, and who take responsibility for the political domain as such (decision making and implementation). In the republican tradition, citizens are the ones who govern and who are being governed (Gunsteren 1992). The traditional virtues were, for example, commitment, sacrifice, discipline, leadership. In neo-republican concepts basic virtues are reason, democratic attitude, deliberation, pluralism (Gunsteren 1992). Radical democracy is another variant, stressing citizenship as sovereignty by the people.

5   Community-based citizenship (Walzer, Etzioni) has its emphasis on the historic developed communities as anchorage for citizens. Social relationships within a community are basically as follows:

> A good society, is one in which people treat one another as ends in themselves and not merely as instruments; as whole persons rather than as fragments; as members of a community, bonded by ties of affection and commitment, rather than only as employers, traders, consumers or even as fellow citizens.

> (Etzioni 2001)

6   Activating citizenship (see Chapters 2 and 3) can be considered as a political strategy to empower citizens and civil society to take responsibility for social, public and private life. Like neo-republicans it defines citizens as agencies who take responsibility for the public domain as well, and that is different from the republican approach, for private life. Citizenship, in this respect, is not merely focusing on individuals but also on society as such. It comes close to the concept of *relational citizenship* that emphasizes citizenship as a practice, a process 'interwoven and transformed over time in all the distinctive and different dimensions of their lives' (Lawy and Biesta 2006). Citizenship in this respect is the outcome and quality of inter-human relationships. It is a continuing learning process in every-day life (Visscher 2008).

Marshall and the discourse on social citizenship

Civil, political and social rights

T. H. Marshall placed social citizenship on the research map of the social sciences through his lecture 'Citizenship and social class' in 1949. Marshall had a sociological way of looking at things and transferred the idea of citizenship from a political into a societal context. Social citizenship was about the relation between the individual and the welfare state he argued, and referred to the citizen as a full member of the community. Social citizenship was based on social rights, providing each individual access to full membership of the community. Marshall's sociological understanding of citizenship implied that he looked upon the social dimension of citizenship as institutionally anchored to the welfare state and welfare system. The normative idea was based on people's need to guarantee citizens a basic security (status), defined in relation to the actual socio-economic context and in the societal social heritage in the meaning of social inequality related to social class. Marshall's concept was related to a vision of creating a decent social basis for all citizens, by providing access to the most elementary social security systems. Above that, each citizen was free to create a higher living standard, in line with the liberal tradition.

Marshall pointed out the history of citizenship, starting with the civil rights, followed by the political rights, developed in the upcoming industrial societies. Civil citizenship was already actualized in the eighteenth century and referred to freedom of speech, thought and faith, the right to own property and to conclude valid contracts, and the right to justice (Marshall and Bottomore 1992: 8) or in the words of President Roosevelt in 1941, 'freedom of speech, freedom of religion, freedom from want, freedom from fear' (Witteveen and Klink 2002). Civil rights were anchored in the judicial system, the courts and laws. Political citizenship was about political rights, such as being politically eligible and having the right to vote. The political rights came up in the nineteenth century and had their institutional basis in the parliamentary and democratic system. Marshall added to the civic and political rights the third dimension of citizenship: social citizenship as connected to and based on the former two. Social citizenship has been developed during the twentieth century. It aimed to guarantee a basic social welfare to all citizens and to create the conditions to get access to their civil and political rights. Social systems, such as education, housing, social security, health and labour are the institutional framework for social citizenship. Civic, political and social rights acting together, promote a further development of contemporary society, Marshall argued. Following Marshall, such co-operation strengthens a sustainable social development of the society.

Reciprocity

The coming together of rights as basic condition for the upcoming welfare state assumes reciprocity as a basic principle. Reciprocity starts from the idea that mutual help and access to common goods is useful for each person. Reciprocity promotes personal interest and shared interest. The weakest degree of reciprocity is the claim of rights, related to the membership of the societal collective: the community, society, state. This collective reciprocity implicates citizenship as including all citizens and was the very basis of Marshall's notion of social citizenship. Therefore, social citizenship is strongly connected to universal social policies. Collective reciprocity is to distinguish three concepts, all of them being selective, in the sense of being directed to and accessible for specific groups of citizens. A first concept of welfare benefits (social rights) is built upon the idea of reciprocity, built on getting back what you have paid before within a national system, for example, public pensions. A second concept is about compensating welfare deficiencies or risks, for example, sickness benefit or disablement allowance. The third concept – basically financial support – is about compensating lack of income and poverty. This third reciprocity is different from the others, because it requests from the person involved to fulfil a number of requirements and duties that are stipulated for getting labour market compensation. Disabled people and people living on social assistance or unemployment benefits are at risk of stigmatization, because of their special position and dependency on collective reciprocity systems. To a certain extent, collective reciprocity substitutes mutual reciprocity within the family or among friends or neighbours. One of the features of the welfare state is freeing citizens from dependency on informal networks in creating more individual autonomy.

Legal and moral rights and duties

Rights are divided into legal and moral rights. Legal rights are based on laws and are enforceable. Most civil and political rights are recorded in laws, a number of them even in constitutions. Social rights are partly legal and partly moral. Legal social rights are, for example, unemployment benefits. Moral rights, often referred to as 'the right to', are not legally based and therefore, more intentional. It is in the order of 'should be'. Moral rights are often interpreted as rights to be guaranteed by the state and to be rooted in the education system, in access to the labour market or housing or in getting social care and social support. The citizen has no enforceable means to get his 'moral' right. Social rights are dependent on political decisions and on economic trends. In periods of recession, entitlements to unemployment benefits and social assistance are under pressure. Another political discourse is on the relationship between rights and duties. The question is whether social rights are guaranteed as such or are dependent on fulfilment of specific duties; for example, access to social assistance or unemployment benefits are related to the obligation to look for a job or to accept voluntary work. Many social rights are in this sense conditional. Marshall's social citizenship and universal rights idea should be reflected from this specific character of social rights and its connection to duties. Marshall did not argue that the aspect of duty was abandoned the whole way through, but there had been a shift from where the citizen has both rights and duties, to emphasizing having rights, he argued (Marshall 1950). In his study *Paying for Social Rights*, Sjöberg (1999) argues that, in contrast to civil and political citizenship, social citizenship is characterized by an extensive societal contribution, based on individual input (taxes, collective insurances) and including wide administrative and distributive systems, which altogether demand big economical recourses (Sjöberg 1999). This economic dimension of social citizenship makes it dependent on the contemporary societal economic context. In that meaning social rights are doubly conditional: first, because they are dependent on public finance, and, second, because only the citizens who have fulfilled their social duties can qualify for them. The importance of social duties has increased in the development of social policy in European welfare states, at the same time as the right to benefits and support has been more limited (Sjöberg 1999).[1] Sjöberg looks critically upon Marshall arguing the shift from conditionally social rights to social rights as such. At least, in recent times, the perspective on the relationship between rights and duties and the volume of social rights are under discussion. Sjöberg notes another direction, opposite to Marshall's perception of the increase of (unconditional) social rights. The shift to the discourse on individual duties and the volume of social rights is going on at the EU level and the European states in a framework where social economic differences are increasing as well (Schierup 2003, 2005). There has been a change of discourse from talking of universal rights at a transnational level towards the talk of moral values, focused on the transition from right to work to duty to work, of the individual, which affects especially migrants' conditions and their social citizenship rights and position in the labour market (Schierup 2003, 2005).

Bottomore: formal and substantial citizenship

Most European debates on migration and citizenship have focused on the formal citizenship – i.e. on the formal regulation for access to citizenship for immigrants, or to become a citizen. Less attention has been paid to substantial citizenship – to be a citizen – i.e. to the actual conditions of and possibilities to exercise your rights and duties, as a 'satisfactory member' of the society, as expressed by Marshall.

(Schierup 2005: 244)

This line of thought is related to what T. Bottomore noted in discussing Marshall's legacy for contemporary multiethnic Europe. Strongly influenced by Marshall, T. Bottomore advanced the citizenship theory further, as discussed by Marshall, by developing the concepts *formal* and *substantial* citizenship. Bottomore discusses the importance of class conflict and social citizenship at a later period than Marshall and therefore in another context. Additionally, he points out the inequality of the substantial social citizenship, related to gender and ethnicity (Bottomore 1992). In a wide understanding, Bottomore discusses social rights in the framework of national health systems, social housing policy, public transport systems and a general access to education. Through the notion of substantial social citizenship Bottomore focuses on the actual functioning of those institutions and people's real access to them. He separates substantial rights from formal citizen rights. Formal citizens' rights are based in the nation state and only partly enforceable and often relate to duties and social competences to get access. Formal citizenship is neither a sufficient nor a necessary prerequisite for substantial citizenship (Bottomore 1992). What really matter are the societal conditions and the personal contexts citizens are in. Social rights hardly have a meaning in very poor countries through lack of institutions and services. Formal rights scarcely count if people live in deprived areas or are confronted with complex situations and the only thing to do is to survive. Even formal rights have no impact if in a social system or in social patterns certain groups are excluded or overlooked, such as women, children, the disabled, or migrants. Substantial citizenship asks for conditions and contexts endorsing social rights and enabling to fulfil social duties. It asks also for clear duties to the state, local authorities, institutions and communities to be accessible and enabling for all citizens. When it comes to women and substantial social rights, according to Bottomore, women have often been discriminated against and still are, in the perspective of having access to the best paid and most prestigious jobs. At the same time the social rights in the societal sections that by tradition have been of special importance for women's full participation, for example, daily child care, parents' insurance and family planning, are more slowly developed than other social services. In the contemporary citizenship discussion, it is for that reason necessary to take into account women's special social position in society, which raises new questions about the extension and content of social rights, Bottomore argues. Extensive migration during the postwar period in Europe has brought about more heterogeneous populations which put new problems and questions in the foreground. It has led to double citizenships and numerous people having only a foreign citizenship. This development brings forward the contemporary role of formal and substantial citizenship rights in the context of migration and multiethnic/cultural societies.

The ethnic perspective

From the ethnic perspective, the reasoning of reciprocity, and rights versus duties leads to further reflections. Are new migrants and certain ethnic communities practically excluded from access to social rights and are there specific duties and demands in integrating into Western societies? Does such a demand even claim assimilation or at least a process of one-way adaptation to the norms and values of the majority? When we come to material (legal) duties, we recognize special ones for migrants in getting national citizenship and residence permits, and in particular in demands related to work. In the domain of moral duties ethnic groups are often perceived as lacking behavioural and educational skills, creating risks for local communities and national societies. Many interventions and moral demands are aimed at specific ethnic groups. Therefore, what are moral duties from an ethnic perspective and how are they perceived by them? In discussing rights and duties, we should reflect on discrimination as well. One of the rights is not to be discriminated against and the reverse side of the coin is the duty to communicate and to deal equally with people with different characteristics. Historically, the most important duty is directed towards the labour market, especially males' participation in the labour market (Sjöberg 1999). It is also where the discrimination primarily occurs. Housing segregation is another area where normative influence has been shown and discriminating practices are to be observed.

From social rights to human rights in the individualized context

Marshall's reasoning was based on the understanding of a welfare state aiming to cover the risks in three main areas – work, war and reproduction – by entitling citizens to social rights. Endorsing production and reproduction was the main reason to establish social rights. This *reproductive citizenship* was basically embedded in the idea of compensation, risk sharing and causality. War invalids or war widows had no guilt for their situation, far from it, and therefore it was reasonable to guarantee a certain income to them. Social rights are universal, in the sense that each citizen in need has the right to support and compensation. The discussion about the entitlement to compensation is still there in societies. One example of causality reasoning is the debate on the status of refugees. In the current debate, asylum seekers (mark the shift from 'refugees' to 'asylum seekers') are often seen as causing their own situation, because they are assumed not be true refugees but seekers of better economic conditions and therefore considered not to be entitled to social rights. Another example – and a very classic one – is about the deserving and undeserving poor. The deserving poor are back on the agenda. Poverty is seen less as a socio-economic mechanism – or institutional embedded phenomenon – and more as a lack of personal competencies, albeit a lack of motivation. Today, the idea of *ontological security* is more stressed. Ontological security seeks the value of human beings in itself, instead of guaranteeing reproduction (Turner 2001). This ontological approach moves from citizens' rights to human rights, reflecting the global society and the decreasing importance of nation states and national citizenship. The notion of rights is becoming more relative and contextual and individualized (Cox 1998). Citizens do not belong explicitly to one society or community but roam through an open, flexible and mobile world. The human rights are implemented in various ways in different places, dependent on the local context. 'Local' implies local communities, as well as international contexts, as institutions, companies and multinationals. In all those places human rights should be the leading norm but the implementation is local. Together with economic restraints, cutting expenses policies and decentralization processes, social rights are becoming more diffuse, vague and diverse. Vulnerable individuals and groups have less clear entitlements and much more difficulty in finding their path through the institutions and local contexts. It creates the risk that social problems can publicly be perceived as personal or related to specific groups. This, in combination with popular and media stigmatizing discourses, can result in discrimination and social exclusion of vulnerable groups (Ålund 2002). Thus, different obstacles in regard to substantial aspects of social citizenship can contribute to accelerate processes of social exclusion, namely blaming the excluded as not fulfilling the duties and demands (Young 2000).

Lister: excluding and including tendency to social citizenship

Citizenship's excluding tendency

Ruth Lister challenges the starting point of Marshall for social citizenship theory, as a *rights discourse*, through criticizing its excluding tendency. She discusses the requirements for an inclusive, subjective social citizenship from a feminist angle. Lister distinguishes two forms of citizenship theory. One is the Marshall inspired, *the liberal*. This tradition is based on an *objective view*, with an apprehension of citizenship as social status, where universal rights are formulated from a rights discourse. In the tradition of the classic liberal citizenship theory, two main arguments for social rights appear: on the one hand they promote the exercise of civil and political rights of groups lacking power and deficient resources. On the other they are required to strengthen individual autonomy. From a feminist point of view, the liberal citizenship theory has been criticized as the reason that the rights are not universal, as implicated in universalism. Though they claim to be universal, the rights are not universal in terms of gender. With the male norm as the basis for the rights discourse, the conditions for social citizenship are different for women and men, and that leads to the social exclusion of women. For that reason, Lister criticizes the liberal model as causing exclusion in terms of gender. The liberal concept does not meet the differentiated needs in social citizenship rights according to women, the disabled and ethnically discriminated or social and economically marginalized groups. Instead, the liberal model inhibits a *false universalism*, she argues.

Lister confronts Marshall's notion of social citizenship with the *civic republican* tradition based on a *subjective view* in the way that the social citizenship is understood as something that you gain through societal participation. The problem with the classic republican approach, Lister argues, is that it is mainly men's traditional acting in the public arena that has been the norm. Citizens in general are agents with a capacity for free choice and self-development, and Lister argues that there is no ground for one gender, the male, to have priority to exercise this capacity. Citizens' agency is performed in a variety of ways and this diversity has to be an integral part of what constitutes the understanding of social citizenship. 'In both liberal and republican traditions the citizen is represented by the abstract, disembodied, individual; the former tradition tries to ignore particularity and the latter to transcend it' (Lister 2003: 71). Profound and essential differences in people's social living are made invisible by this lack of context. From a feminist angle it is argued that both traditions' excluding tendency should be met through reformulating social citizenship, not just by adding women as a group, but by including them. Recognition of women's specific conditions and needs is demanded when forming the normative base of social citizenship. The satisfactory social citizenship is based neither on women's similarities with men nor on the differences from men, but instead it ought to be constructed as a *gender-inclusive* citizenship (Lister 2003: 116). In this line of thought, Lister suggests balancing the public and private domain in the concept of citizenship. By leaving out the private arenas, women have a weaker position by definition and by leaving out the private sphere, essential aspects in social citizenship are overlooked. Feminist citizenship theory explains differences in the women's and men's divergent representation in the public arena, which is the one that primarily qualifies for social rights. The question of equal circumstances is also a question of possibilities to act on equal terms. Universalism gets a new dimension, similar to the underlying issue of autonomy. Women's autonomy becomes a necessary requirement for the actual universalism of citizenship policy and seems essential in Lister's reasoning. Autonomy cannot just be seen from an individualistic perspective; it has a broader meaning. It implies a social dimension of power and actualizes the fact that women are often economically dependent on others that limits their possibilities for a satisfactory social citizenship. On one hand you find women to a lesser extent than men in the public arena. On the other hand women are to a greater extent than men actors in the private sphere. Women therefore do not have the chance to qualify for social rights on equal conditions as men because care work and the private arena – according to the male perspective – do not qualify for similar social rights and do not count for satisfactory participation in the public spheres. In this way, the *false universalism* of actual social citizenship acts to exclude women from citizenship rights (Lister 1997, 2003, 2007). While discussing the issue of citizenship from an excluding perspective, Lister elaborates on two perspectives: exclusion *from within* and *from without*. Exclusion, Lister argues, appears in the public and private arenas in society. The public arenas are characterized by the idea of production and political power and are foremost male fields of acting. Exclusion and inclusion in relation to social citizenship describes more a continuum of participation, rather than an absolute dichotomy (Lister 1997, 2003). Through the exclusion tendency of social citizenship, internationally as well as nationally, people are totally or partly excluded from public arenas as well as from private arenas. In this situation the two categories are shaped, those who are *excluded from without* since they do not get access into the country, for instance, asylum seekers migrants. In this group women form a significant proportion (Lister 1997). The other category is those who are *excluded from within*, from an inside position, meaning they live in a society without access to a satisfactory social citizenship. While de-constructing the unitary social category of women, patterns of intersectional exclusion step forward. In this process, class, race, disability, sexuality and age interact (Lister 1997).

Difference and universalism

Lister tries to combine the advantages of a universal approach, including all people, and diversity, referring to the specific groups and positions they are in. To claim for the particularity, it supports social participation of disadvantaged groups in a structural way. The relationship between the universal, selective and particular has been defined by S. Thompson and P. Hoggett (1996). The authors relate particularity to positive selectivity. Positive selectivity is directed towards discriminated groups and is meant to strengthen their position. A social policy in that direction should be regarded as a supplement to the universal expressed in the words of Thompson and Hoggett: 'deliberately abstracts form differences between persons and groups in order to treat all of them fairly' (Thompson and Hoggett 1996: 33). Positive selectivity is different from particularity, Thompson and Hogget argue. Particularity recognizes a group's own conditions and claims. Positive selectivity can be pacifying while particularity is activating by empowering interventions: 'There is a close affinity between particularise and empowerment' (Thompson and Hoggett 1996: 32). In this vein, Young has challenged the discourse with her pledge for a differentiated social citizenship. In the discussion of *politics of difference* (Young 1990, 2000) she claims the recognition of difference and the special needs of vulnerable groups, asking for provision of 'special group' rights. The criticisms directed towards such a differentiated and targeting policy is at risk of strengthening group identities and the interests of certain groups. More targeting policies can endanger more universal approaches or create competition among different interest groups.

The discussion on social citizenship as an excluding and including phenomenon could be seen as leading to a crossroads, with the choice between the different traditions *liberal* and *civic republican* also between the standpoints for universalism or differentiation. The tension occurs in the contradiction of the excluding tendency of citizenship in relation to the promise of inclusion implicated in universal citizenship. However, recent research has rather challenged such tensions by searching for forms of more inclusive citizenship, based in the understanding of the diverse conditions and needs of different groups. An inclusive citizenship holds respect for cultural diversity as well as for formal rights, that comprises both acceptance of universal principles and acknowledgement of diversity (Lister 2007). Searching for what can be the link between universalism and particularism appears to be crucial in the ongoing debate. 'The problematic issue in the current debate is about the universalism (constituting the core of the classic sociological citizenship theory) and the claim to an acknowledgement of differences that combat division and practices of exclusion which appear as differences' (Ålund (2005: 293) with reference to Lister (2006)).

Lister's notion of *differentiated universalism* seems to go beyond the universal and particular dichotomy. Lister addresses, in this notion, the liberal idea of free and equal rights for all citizens but also for an understanding of each citizen or groups, as different in its own right as active agents, in relation to both the private and the public arenas (Lister 1997, 2003). The way for feminist theory to go, Lister argues, is to perceive citizenship from both perspectives, social citizenship as status as well as agency to achieve an inclusive *and* universal citizenship. The criticism of excluding social citizenship and false universalism does not imply abandoning the aim of universal citizenship.

With the concept of *differentiated universalism* she argues for a synthesis of social rights, political participation and civic agency. It is an attempt to combine the core of citizenship as universal, with a policy of difference. The crucial idea is that real universalism can be achieved only when differences are included (Lister 1997, 2003). Limited social citizenship (in formal and substantial aspects) should be met through differentiated universalism, which Lister characterizes as the meeting point between universalism and particularism. 'Tension can be creative, pointing the way to what we might term a "differentiated universalism" in which the achievement of the universal is contingent upon attention to difference' (Lister 2003: 91). Lister seeks the possibility to create conditions for a satisfactory social citizenship to all groups of citizens by looking at the diverse needs which appear and in making diversity an integral part of the norm of social citizenship. Instead of just *adding* diverse needs and differences related to specific groups, they must be *included* as a profound element in the universal social citizenship. She focuses especially on the private care sphere. The idea behind a *differentiated universalism* is to form a universal citizenship that is based on differences within social categories as gender, class, ethnicity, disabilities, sexual preferences and age. The relation between the two dimensions of social citizenship – status and practice – is formed by the agency of the citizen in social and political arenas. In such an interaction between the social and political citizenship, it will be possible for women to strengthen their positions in the society. It will happen when social rights and duties in reality – or in their implementation – create require-ments needed for political agency of each citizen, and this in turn is necessary to extend and uphold social citizenship (Lister 2003). This is the point where conditions for activating citizenship come into focus as will be discussed in the next section.

Activating citizenship within the welfare state

The discourse on social citizenship from Marshall to Lister got its political answer in *activating citizenship* as a driving concept in recent European discussions. The perceptions on activating citizenship differ greatly. Opponents challenge the neo-liberal attempt to undermine social citizenship, in particular by bringing back the substance of social rights. Others support activating citizenship as bridging the gaps between the different political ideologies and opening a common basis for European unification. Activating citizenship became popular at the end of the twentieth century. The sudden rise of unemployment in the early 1980s called for drastic interventions and one of them was to focus on participation in the labour market, more than safeguarding social rights. Income through work – the work, work, work – was the European policy. Labour participation widened under pres-sure, for example, from the feminist angle to participation in labour, care and civil society. From more political arenas, political participation was brought in. Activating citizenship became the overarching concept for the different participa-tion issues. By this, the social rights perspective disappeared from the foreground in this respect that social rights were brought into connection with the participation paradigm. A social society asks for participating citizens in different fields and from there social rights can be safeguarded and guaranteed.

Critical debates about social and activating citizenship

In the political arena, activating citizenship is broadly accepted and proclaimed by management in day-to-day speech. In the social discourse we find a more ambiguous point of view. In principle, the idea of a socially committed citizen responsible for his or her own living and working conditions is not the issue. However, we find a number of objections and considerations.

1   As seen in the Marshall discourse, social citizenship as a universal principle can bring about exclusion because a number of citizens are not able to meet the social duties and access the social resources. This argument is even more valid for activating citizenship. In the European discourses, recognition of diversity, contextuality, differentiation and balancing between universal and targeting policies is essential to realize activating and social citizenship.

2   Activating citizenship is often felt by citizens as an over-demanding and overcharging concept. Vulnerable citizens, informal carers, volunteers and street-level social professionals get the feeling that they are underachieving. Activating citizenship can be used for misjudging the efforts made by so many carers and socially responsible citizens. The most important principle in activating citizenship is that each person *to his or her own capacities* tries to meet the ideal of active citizenship. The second one is to recognize that some citizens are strong in political participation, others in labour, in caring, in civil society, in informal initiatives and relationships. Many efforts in activating citizenship in so-called marginal groups or ethnic minorities are overlooked by standardized monitoring procedures.

3   We find a certain tension between political, civil and social rights. Political rights are partly protective rights against the state and other public agencies, who intervene too much in private life. Other political and civil rights are asking protection of citizens by the state. And social rights are asking for resources from the state. Those different demands in rights from the state are bridgeable but fragile. Current pressing issues are, for example, privacy and the fight against terrorism, or privacy and the entitlement to social assistance.

4   In the concept of activating citizenship it is unclear who exactly is responsible for what. The whole discourse is on shared responsibility between the public, private (family, individual, etc.), civil society and the market sector, as well as between global, regional, national and local levels. Who is responsible for getting people into work if jobs are not available: the market, the public sector, civil society? The risk is that activating citizenship is just a political mission without any implementing power. The enabling state needs hands and feet to create the substance for an active civil society and citizens as main social agencies.

5   In social citizenship and activating citizenship the focus is on the citizen, and rights and duties for citizens. Essential in the discourse is mirroring the debate, opening the discussion about rights and duties for the state and public sector to enable material and substantial social citizenship.

Discussion and assignments

Discussion

- How important is civil society for the functioning of the state? Give reasons.
- Discuss Bottomore's statement about formal and substantial citizenship. He stresses the fact that rights as such are not a guarantee of realized citizenship. What is substantial citizenship asking from society and the state?
- What is your opinion about activating citizenship? Can you give some arguments in favour of activating citizenship and some against it?
- Do you agree with Ruth Lister? What is attractive about her argument?

Assignment 1

Investigate some history on citizenship and civil society in your country and relate it to the overview in this chapter.

Assignment 2

Investigate the national policy in the domain of citizenship and civil society. Are there documents, debates, laws about those issues in your country?

4 Social work under construction

Introduction

In this chapter we will discuss the impact of the transformation and integration process on social work and social professionals. The chapter starts with an overview of some of the basics: the concept, the meanings, the roots and the theories. The second section is on the impact of the transformation on the concept, the position and embedment of social work and the most important tasks. The third section is more on the technical issues, such as methodology and competences in social work. The chapter concludes with a reflection on the social professional in citizenship-based social work.

Clarifying the basics

Social work as a broad concept

Since the last few decades it is popular to use *social work* as an overall term for the different social professions, defining social work as 'a network of occupations' (Payne 2005). It is a broader concept than social work used to be. Using the English terms 'social work' all over Europe indicates the international dimension. There is a certain urgency to create a common recognized and accepted term and concept for the field social professionals are in. Overall in Europe, hundreds of different professions and functions have been created in care and welfare provision. In contrast with nurses, policemen or doctors, social professionals are hardly recognizable because of the lack of a common name and accepted body of knowledge (Thole 2002a). It seems a fragmented world with rather vague objectives and unclear outcomes (Dominelli 2004, Banks 2006). Therefore, many social experts felt the need for a more shared concept and a common ground for all professionals in the different domains in the social sector. We have to overcome fragmentation and confusion. A third argument for employing social work as an overarching concept is the fact that in social practice we have to put up with blurring borders between the different social professions. Studies have learnt that most professional competences in the different social professions are rather similar and comparative (Thole 2002b, Lorenz 2006, Payne 2006). The next argument for broadening the scope is the international trend to foster employability.

Employability implies that professionals are continuing learning and self-improving and regularly change their positions in a broad professional domain. It is suggested that too narrowly educated professionals are caught and cannot escape their own specialty, being too competent in too small a domain. Therefore, broad domains and basically broad professional parameters offer employers and employees better opportunities for development. A final argument is to be found in the European Bologna Declaration on first degree and Masters course structure of higher education. Undergraduate degree courses in particular suggest a broad orientation on a certain professional and a certain scientific, or knowledge, domain. For those reasons social work as an overall label has become popular but disputed at the same time. Social workers in the more traditional sense fear diffusion about their profession and social pedagogues have difficulties in identifying themselves as social workers. Other experts do not agree with the broad concept at all because it is too broad and imprecise in their opinion. One of the alternatives to consider is to introduce social professional instead of social worker as the overarching term (Lyons *et al.* 2006). It prevents the confusion about the different concepts of social work and it recognizes the umbrella character and does not suggest that all the different social professions are brought back to one profession. If somebody is asking what your profession is, the answer could be 'I am a social professional', or more particularly, 'I am a social worker, or a social pedagogue, or a community worker, or an art therapist, or a care consultant, etc.'.

Different meanings of social work

We should be well aware of the fact that social work has different meanings. Reading about social work means always to understand which perspective is meant by the author and unfortunately many authors are quite imprecise in this respect. Social work has at least four different meanings (Ewijk 2009):

1   Social work as a field of activities. Social work stands for a certain sector or branch and partly covers concepts as *social services* and *social welfare* or *(social) care and welfare*. Nationally and internationally we are lacking transparent concepts. Social work in this first meaning can be seen as an overall term for all services, activities and provisions in social welfare or the care and welfare sector. It is a common field of social action (Scherr 2002, Payne 2005).

2   Social work as a professional domain. It comprises all professions in social welfare. The debate here is whether we are only referring to professionals as higher educated professionals or are including all care and welfare workers with different levels of education. Another debate is about what professions belong to the social professions. Borders are blurred, with professions in health and education (Payne 2005, Lyons *et al.* 2006).

3   Social work is a highly specialized profession, which has a common standard, common ethics, common codes, a centralized registration and permanent professionalization. Social work in the UK, for instance, had much of those

characteristics. It was a profession within or very close to the public sector and mainly operating in the field of social assistance to people in marginal positions and multi-problem contexts. Casework was seen as the basic method of social work (Jones 2002).

4   Social work as a common field of social action, social theories and social work research or the social work body of knowledge. Most European universities have created undergraduate and Masters courses in social work, departments of social work and appointed social work professors and teachers. Social work as a discipline and science is nevertheless debated. Social professionals bring together different scientific disciplines, such as psychology, sociology, pedagogy, law and public/social administration, and connect those theories with social actions and practical experience. Therefore the body of knowledge of social work is highly complicated, and different from the 'traditional' discipline orientation of most universities but very challenging and interesting and could be seen as one of the most intriguing scientific fields of studying human behaviour, human relationships and social systems (Thole 2002a, Keller 2005).

In this book *social work* refers to the social work body of knowledge, including all social professions. *Social professions* and *social professionals* stand for professionals with higher first degrees and higher degrees in social welfare.

Different roots

Social professions have different roots and the traditions are different from country to country. Bringing this all together, six different roots of social professions can be distinguished (Ewijk *et al.* 2007).

> Social work has a long tradition in case work and orientation on citizens who – temporally – need social assistance and social support. It basically focuses on problem solving considering the material problems (debts, income, job), the individual problems (lack of certain competences, disabilities and impairments, socio psychological problems) and contextual problems (family life, ethnic backgrounds, informal networks, communities).
>
> (Jones 2002)

> Social education and social pedagogy. Both terms are not fully similar to each other but the main perspective is on the (social) development of people, in particular children and youth. It is often seen as oriented on upbringing and family life, sometimes even offering a substitute 'family life' in institutions, foster families, small units in neighbourhoods, childcare and daycare centres. On the other hand social education refers to the social context of upbringing and social development. It is about the configuration of school, family, youth and childcare, leisure time activities and the more physical environment (ecologic pedagogy). Social education has its main focus

on children and youth but it definitely regards adults as well. Social development does not halt at the age of 18 or 25! In each stage of life people have to prepare for the next stage and to accept and to adapt to the stage they are in. Sometimes professional support is needed to make the transitions properly.

(Niemeyer 2002)

Psychology and psychiatry. In many countries psychology and psychologists are partly integrated in social professions. In youth care and mental healthcare social workers and psychologists meet and compete with each other. In new professions specializing in diagnosis, indication and assessments psychologists and social workers are often found in the same jobs. The influence of psychology, psychiatry and clinical social work on the body of knowledge of social work is immense.

Community work. Community workers are focused on empowering and supporting communities, mostly territorially based communities, like the neighbourhood, a small village or a district in the big cities. Community workers sometimes manage a community centre and the activities in it. Other community workers are more focused on supporting and strengthening social actions and social cohesion in neighbourhoods. Mostly, community workers work with groups and projects, quite often in the field of socio-cultural activities (for example, community art) and sporting activities, mostly outside the formal sport clubs.

(Smith 2006)

Community development. Community development is close to community work. Its roots are however much more in community-based work in developing countries. Community development includes all aspects of life, like setting up schools, health centres, a local administration, water supplies and roads. In community development the focus is currently on strengthening civil society as well. The locals have to organize their own communities and should be supported by experts and not the other way round.

(Ferguson and Dickens 1999, Keller 2003)

Social care. Social care is generally identified as care for people with disabilities and frail elderly people. Quite often care for homeless people, mental health users, youth care and childcare are included as well. The emphasis is on support and delivery of services and care products. Social care covers long-term care as well as home care and community care. Nurses and low or not educated care workers for cleaning, washing, meals, etc. have for long dominated this field. In the care for the learning disabled many social pedagogues were and are employed. Recently, all kinds of social professionals are more involved in social care because of community care, the growing number of people in need of care and because of the increasing complexities in social care due to de-institutionalization. Another change in this field is the shift from a more cure and medical approach to a more care and activation strategy. This asks for a different kind of professional as well and is sometimes felt as threatening social work professionalism, changing the profession in a more caring one.

(Cree 2002, Dominelli 2004)

Socio-art therapy and community art. It is debatable whether socio- and art therapists on the one hand and community art on the other, belong to the social professions. It is argued that socio- and art therapists are in between health and social work and more focused on counselling, empowering, guiding and less on curing and diagnostic activities. In different European countries undergraduate and postgraduate degree courses cover these sorts of therapists and community (art) workers as well. In particular, art therapists and social cultural workers have social work enriched with the power of using media, like music, drama and modern communication technology. Those 'techniques' empower people and communities, appeal to their creative capacities and contribute to connecting people.

Different theories

We find different opinions and discourses about the essential perspective in social work. There are different 'schools' in the social work domain (Bouverne and Ewijk 2008). The broadly accepted 'official' social work Montreal definition (see p 68) stands for promoting 'social change, problem solving in human relationships and the empowerment and liberation of people to enhance wellbeing' (Hare 2004). Payne makes a comparable claim for social work. 'It is this: that social improvement can be achieved by interpersonal influence and action, that social change can be harnessed to individual personal development and that carrying out these two activities together should be a profession' (Payne 2006: 1). Maybe the Montreal definition and Payne's claim are covering social work broadly. However, behind those statements we find many different positions, perspectives and approaches in social work. In this overview section, it is impossible to deal extensively with this highly interesting discourse on social work theory, but to give some indication about different points of view, some of the most significant perspectives will be discussed very shortly.

Social work as task-centred work

In this approach, strongly based in the Anglo Saxon tradition, we perceive social work as a preventive, short term intervention with a strong methodical and technical approach. The first step is to identify – in dialogue with the user – a concrete problem. The next step is to design a plan to solve the problem, usually with some more material aspects (benefit, access to the labour market, debt relief) and some immaterial support, for example, five counselling sessions. After short term intervention, the process will be evaluated. In case work methodology peer supervision is an important element. In peer supervision, cases are discussed and compared, and it is sometimes referred to as practice-based learning. Evidence, effect, efficiency are important criteria to apply in case work methodology. The short term intervention approach is open for designing and applying protocols, sometimes highly prescriptive (Doel 2002).

Constructive social work

This approach has its roots in the Anglo Saxon tradition as well, and is quite the opposite of the strong methodical and technical approach, starting from the presumption that an objective reality does not exist but we live in a constructed, ever changing world and that all observations are about perception and language (Parton 1996, Parton *et al.* 2007). In this respect social work is not a scientific technical methodology to solve problems but more supportive to people in their continuing search to cope with life, and to create a certain identity. De-construction and co-construction are popular concepts, referring to the fact that it is important to be aware of the constructiveness of realities and perceptions and the necessity to 'break through' one's own perceptions and to create a new openness in coping with situations and contexts the person is in. Co-construction is the process to arrive at new perceptions and solutions by a process of interaction, for example, between user and social worker. A social worker is somebody who goes along with the user, is open and supportive, is creative and constructive. Much importance is given to telling stories, poems and narratives: 'Whereas science looks for explanation and causes, the story of narrative approach is intent to find a *meaningful* account' (Parton 2002: 243).

Managerialism

A third approach, recently strong, again, in the Anglo Saxon world, is greatly influenced by a businesslike approach to social work, stressing the consumer position of the user. A user is someone with a need or question looking for a service, in kind or in person, to help him or her. The social professional is someone who is not interpreting the need of the user but answering it. Social professionals are delivering services, such as counselling, information, practical support and coaching. Managerialism is related to an increasing involvement of the private sector and its emphasis on choice, efficiency and evidence (Cree 2002). Along with managerialism and market orientation is an approach to strengthen the user position, not only as a customer but also as someone to have a say in the process of service provision, and even in the education of social workers.

Social pedagogy

In the section on 'roots' we introduced social pedagogy as having continental European roots. Because it has often been compared and contrasted with social work, we come back to the special perspective of social pedagogy. Social pedagogy starts from the assumption that human beings become human beings (Niemeyer, 2002) only through communities ('Gemeinschaft'). It is focused on societal processes and tries to support people in their own community. Concepts such as social cohesion, social capital, and in particular, social competences are currently leading in this tradition. Group work, community work and individual social work are seen as different aspects in the process of social educating. Seen from this point of view, social work is more about a semi-structural 'service' in communities to support individuals, groups and communities in social relationships and competences than a client-concentrated intervention. Clubs, youth centres, community centres, supporting volunteering work, counselling parents, children, people in need, are at the heart of social pedagogy. On the European continent the social pedagogy approach has been and still is often dominant. In many countries, for example, Denmark, France, Switzerland, the Netherlands, social work and social pedagogy are seen as separate areas. However, recently social work and social pedagogy are coming together more. In Germany, social pedagogy and social work are brought together in the education system (Thole 2002a). The exciting issue is the question of whether the continental mix of social work (in its restricted sense) and social pedagogy creates a different perspective and approach from the broader Anglo Saxon social work concept.

Critical social work

Critical social work – continental and Anglo Saxon originated – places social work in the macro-economic system and discourse. It analyses the dependency of social professions on the financiers and the national and local authorities in the public sector. Social work in this critical perspective is regarded as being about disciplining people, teaching them to adapt to their social positions. Critical social work in the 1970s was about solidarity with the working class and about developing an awareness that they were exploited by the capitalist system (Deppe 1973). And some authors hope for a revival:

> This approach is grounded in an analysis of capital – following Marx – and the authors believe that it is time for this to find its way back on to the social work agenda, by bringing to the fore an analysis that shows how recent transformations have sought to mask the economic realities of 21st-century capitalism.
>
> (Price and Simpson 2007: 6)

After the Marxist period in critical social work, critical social work identified itself with the emancipating processes of different groups, such as women, the poor, immigrants and children, looking at society as a creator of categories, problems, exclusion and disabilities (Barnes *et al.* 2002).

Anti-oppressive social work

Anti-oppressive social work tries to support people and liberate them from processes in their life, hindering a fair development and access to the social systems (education, health, labour market, social security, housing). In the words of Lena Dominelli, 'Eradicating oppression and asserting their right to self-expression in a world that they control has become a key concern of peoples across the globe' (2002a: 1). Therefore, she argues, promoting social justice and human development in an unequal world provides the 'raison d'être' of social work practice. Anti-oppressive social work addresses social divisions and structural inequalities in the work that is done with clients. Power is one of the essential concepts in this approach. Dominelli discriminates between *power over* as dominance, and *power to* as the potential to take action, and *power of* as the collective strength to achieve a common object. She emphasizes the transformative power, the power to change by combining the power to and power of and fighting the power over (Dominelli 2002b). Anti-oppressive work is therefore also 'a methodology focusing on both process and outcome and a way of structuring relationships between individuals that aims to empower users by reducing negative effects of hierarchy in their immediate interaction and the work they do together' (Dominelli 2002b: 6). The anti-oppressive perspective is rooted in the 1960s (Freire) and critical social work. Nowadays there is strong awareness of the risk of social work becoming oppressive by focusing on issues of control (Dominelli 2002a, Smith 2002).

Faith-based social work

(Inter) Faith-based social work has its roots and inspiration in religion. It believes that human life and human understanding is embedded in spirituality and the profound connection with the environment (Canda 1998). Actually, religious and spiritual factors have often been linked more to pathology and impediments rather than seen as strengths of resources in a client's situation (Zapf 2005). Between social workers from the different world religions, such as Islam, Hinduism, Buddhism, Judaism and Christianity, is a common understanding that belief, meaningfulness, dignity, reconciliation, harmony, family and community are basic elements for social workers and their clients. In this respect, faith-based social work criticizes the dominant Western social work approach with it emphasis on change, remedial approaches, self-responsibility, individualism and the focus on the state and rights (Ferguson 2005). They feel in the 'human and social rights' debate a neglect of the real situations in poor countries and they want to start with much more of a need orientation, answering the needs of the very poor (Ife and Fiske 2006). Within this approach a more critical voice is heard, stating that Western social workers are too professionalized and 'technical' and have lost their commitment to fighting for social justice and the poor.

We can wonder if the choice of one of the theories should be left to the social professional or social services. The different theories affect substantially the social professional approach. It makes a difference if the user is seen from the faith-based social work theory or anti-oppressive one, from a constructive or managerial approach. It seems confusing for citizens and financiers if the approach differs from professional to professional. Mostly, social professionals and social services are not outspoken about their perception on social problems, users and theories. At the heart of social work we meet these problematic questions. Who decides? What theory is chosen or are we mixing them in a melting pot? How free is each professional to commit themselves to one or two theories and what does this mean for the users and the perception of social work as a profession?

The impact of the transformation

Privatization, strengthening civil society, localization and integration are changing the landscape and are challenging social work and social professionals to answer to the changes.

The classic division in the social professions between social workers, social pedagogues, social care workers, community workers, and socio- and art therapists is not clearly defined and under discussion. Social welfare is expanding and/or threatened, particularly in the grey areas between social welfare and healthcare and social welfare and education (Cree 2002). Social work as a body of knowledge is challenged by new perspectives and changing populations. We shall discuss the definition, positions, competences and core tasks for an adequate social work.

Citizenship-based social work

Regarding the transformation from the welfare state into an activating state and the impact on the social domain, in particular on the social services, a repositioning of the social services and the social professionals is urgent. The 'Montreal' definition of social work is as follows:

> The social work profession promotes social change, problem solving in human relationships, and the empowerment and liberation of people to enhance wellbeing. Utilizing theories of human behaviour and social systems, social work intervenes at the points where people interact with their environments. Principles of human rights and social justice are fundamental to social work.
>
> (IFSW 2009a)

The declaration is an attempt to adapt the profession of social work to modern society. The strength of this definition is the fact that it is agreed upon by experts representing different countries and positions and by the Federation of Social Workers and the Schools of Social Work. It implies a certain weakness at the same time. Its first problem is that it does not really cover the other roots and theories of the social professions, such as social pedagogy and social care. The definition expands former social work definitions rather than creating a new umbrella definition embracing the whole family of social professions. Its second 'problem' is the emphasis on words such as wellbeing and liberation, lacking an appeal to current social policies and representing an overestimation of social work capacity. The whole definition has the risk of being associated with a left-wing political position, a good corner to be in as a citizen, but risky for a profession.

The transformation creates a new challenge and opportunity to reposition social workers at the heart of social policies. Socio-cultural concepts are closer to social work and social education than macro socio-economic politics. The emphasis on civil society, activation and participation is referring to classic assignments for social professionals. Localization and its contextual and integrative concept foster the idea of a social professional with a more holistic and process oriented connotation. Privatization has a more ambiguous effect on the development of social professionals. It creates new markets and a new profile connected with entrepreneurship. In this respect it enriches the profession. On the other hand it economizes the social domain and turns users into consumers and social work into products and services. Overseas experiences learn that a kind of social dumping in the professional domain is affected by privatization. Low qualified care workers will carry out most of the work. The multicultural reality changes attitudes and approaches and emphasizes bridging and de-constructing qualities of social professionals. It enriches the workforce with social professionals from other backgrounds and it adds new dimensions to social work and social education. I suggest therefore the next definition: 'Citizen-based social work, as a field of action, knowledge and research, aims at integration of all citizens, and supports and encourages self-responsibility, social responsibility and the implementation of social rights' (Ewijk 2009). Here, integration in society and community, citizenship, responsibility and social rights are key words. It is not a discussion about words only. Its impact is on accepting concepts such as activating citizenship, activating state and social work as a common domain for research, action and knowledge. Social work in this sense is a normative profession based on a concept of citizenship as expressed in the section above. It is most important to stress that social support has always been in the hands of citizens and should be in future as well. Social services and social professionals are additional and try to strengthen and support individuals and their informal networks and not to replace them. The citizen-based social fabric sometimes needs professional support, for example, in information, consultancy, training, intervention, delivery of homecare services, shelter, enabling social action and social cohesion. Social work aims at enabling, supporting, strengthening citizens, their networks and communities. It is not the 'cure department'. Social work as science and the social profession should start from the assumption that citizens are able to cope with their own lives and collective life but sometimes individuals, groups or communities need additional support because they cannot cope properly any more with their lives, and professional support and intervention is necessary.

Three or four corners

In the introduction I presented the Payne triangle (Figure 0.1, p. 2), suggesting transforming it into a square. Here we find social work categorized in three different basic methodological approaches and related to their ideological positioning (see Figure 0.2, p. 3).

The first corner is the *reflexive-therapeutic* one, where clients gain power over their own feelings and way of life, and where they achieve personal growth, self-actualization and personal power over their environment. It relates to psycho-dynamic, humanist, extentialist, constructive and crisis interventions (Payne 2002, 2005). It helps people to understand themselves and their relationships better and to move on to a more effective way of dealing with their situation (Dominelli 2002b).

Socialist-collectivist is in the next corner, and according to Payne, 'The most oppressed and disadvantaged people can gain power over their lives' (2005: 10). Emancipatory approaches or transformational ones such as critical, anti-oppression, feminist and empowerment, are in the foreground. Dominelli collects those approaches under the heading 'emancipatory approaches' and characterizes them as having an explicit commitment to social justice and engagement in overt challenges to the welfare system (Dominelli 2002b).

Individualist reformist is in the third corner. Payne is quite concise in explaining this corner, stating that it is about maintaining the social order. Characteristic approaches are social development, system oriented approaches, cognitive-behavioural and task centred. Maybe we should add 'punitive social work' in recognition of justice related approaches, being tough on illegal migrants, the unemployed and anti-social behaviour among (young) people (Smith 2002, Dominelli 2004, Hayes and Humphries 2006).

Contextual-transformational could be the fourth corner. In this corner citizenship-based social work is the perspective. Activating individuals, networks and communities is in the foreground. Participation, strengthening social capital (relationships, trust) and social competences are characteristic of this approach. The focus is on changing situations, improving contexts, strengthening relationships (Ewijk 2007, 2009).

Three basic positions

Social professionals are differently positioned in social work and social policy. The position is another defining factor. I distinguish three main positions.

1   *Front line workers.* Front line social professionals work on the local level and intermingle in the social life of the locals. Their core task is to activate people and neighbourhoods and to support the most vulnerable citizens. Sometimes interventions are needed to solve problematic situations or conflicts and tense relationships within a family, a group or the whole community. Front line workers work together with citizens and together with professionals from other fields, like education, health, housing, police and local authorities. Front line workers are 'neighbourhood watchers' or the eyes, ears, hands, heart and brains in the neighbourhood together with the local residents. They initiate social actions, in particular by addressing institutions and local authorities. Front line

workers are found in community work, in social (case) work, in social pedagogy and in social care.

2   *Entrepreneurs.* The rising private market of the social services creates a new profile for social workers. The need for innovators, managers, account managers, designers and developers of successful product and market combinations, care consultants and social entrepreneurship in social care, child care, youth care, socio-cultural activities, community art, sports is growing quickly. More social services are becoming businesses and ask for a business oriented attitude. Market-driven social services can provide luxury arrangements, special treatments, innovation projects and all kinds of care services directly available for consumers or purchased by local authorities or insurance companies.

3   *Specialists.* A third option for social workers can be found in the position of a specialist with expertise in a certain method, a specific target group or a special field of activities, for example, youth care institutions, nursing homes for dementia, day care centres for people with learning difficulties. Specialists are trained in particular for a specified function (for example, diagnosis and assessment), a specific method (video home training) or specific field of activities (for example, youth care rehabilitation centre).

Core tasks

There are many lists of core tasks, qualifications and competences in social professions. The list presented here is only a tentative one and reflects the impact of the transformation. We should expect that social professionals are competent to carry out the next seven core tasks.

1   To implement social rights and duties by information, consultation and referral. Social professionals operate quite often as counsellors and guides. They need professional knowledge about the different laws and regulations and provisions in social welfare and neighbouring sectors (education, housing, etc.) and professional knowledge about backgrounds and characteristics of their users. Counselling services for families, youngsters or elderly people belong to these core tasks. Of course, the techniques and methods of listening, explaining and consulting are needed. It should be borne in mind that activating social rights is two-sided: the user has his or her obligations and the providers of education have theirs too. Social professionals have to bridge both sides and aim at improvements on both sides.

2   To activate people to take care of their own living and working conditions and their own behaviour. Social professionals are expected to have the capacity and competence to influence people's behaviour, relationships and contexts. In many cases a certain change in behaviour and/or attitude is critical in improving the situation. The request to change behaviour is not always demanded by users themselves. Often other people or other professionals are asking social professionals to help them get people back to

work or school. Apart from activation as a temporary support and intervention, some people need lifelong support to be a full citizen, as we have seen under 'contextual citizenship'.

3   To endorse and promote social responsibility and social cohesion. Maybe even more complicated is the task to change and improve relationships between relatives, between neighbours, between different groups of local residents, between different ethnic groups, etc. Generally, the change is asked for by one of the actors, hoping that the social professional is able to change the other actor. Professionals usually opt for change in the whole pattern of social relationships, not focusing on just one of the actors. It is about the bridging qualities of social professionals, bridging between people, bridging between people and institutions, between citizens and society.

4   To support developing social competences. In particular social educators or social pedagogues are often involved in education and training programmes for all kinds of groups. The broad social development and social education assignment in social welfare has been partly displaced by more problem oriented policies. Partly social development tasks are passed on to the education institutions. With the shift to more socio-cultural approaches and in empowering local communities this more personal development-based core task is definitely back on the social work agenda.

5   To manage care. A social professional is able to manage care for a certain person or group of people. The professional is not directly carrying out care services but organizing care, evaluating care and sometimes providing some complex care tasks. In particular in the fields of elderly care, care management, youth care and care consultancy are fast growing 'markets' open to social professionals.

6   To intervene in to and answer to individual, group and community problems. The social professional reflex should be to activate and support people, institutions, and to take action. Naturally, if needed – and it is often needed – social professionals intervene and react directly and personally to social needs of users. The direct client contacts and interaction will always be an essential part in social professions.

7   To supervise and control. Most social professionals have a strong tendency to help people, to assist them, to represent their interests, to act as advocates for them. However, many politicians and policy makers and 'the public' expect social professionals to keep things and people in control, to intervene in serious conflicts, to fight criminality, to promote social safety in neighbourhoods. We certainly find an increasing emphasis on this side of social welfare. Social professionals should accept and adopt this core task in many cases.

The meta-methodology of social work[1]

This section is on the methodological basis of social work. We discriminate between a basic methodology being essential for all social professionals and specific methods connected to specific professions and specific tasks. However, there are two warnings. A description of a method looks very systematic and can create the impression of a mechanical application. However, in reality things are often confusing, changing and different steps in a methodology are interactive. The whole planning circle should be gone round several times during a project or intervention. The second warning is that a basic methodology needs to adapt and to be transferred to the specific context. The basic methodology is applicable to working with individuals, with groups and communities but needs transformation in all of those cases. It is up to a professional to tailor it. In the framework of this book, it was not possible and adequate to make an investigation and categorization of the thousands of methods and instruments in social work practice.

Explanation of basic terminology

Methodology of a profession

Professional methodology is a specified and systematic way of carrying out the professional tasks and activities that is basically recognized and recognizable for the professionals in that profession. Characteristic of a methodology is that it is explained and written down. The methodology is also systematic, logical and relevant. It supports professionals in working effectively and transparently. A professional applies the methodology on a daily basis, quite often rather automatically, as it becomes a habit.

A method

A method is a specified and systematic way to achieve a defined objective. The definition has common elements with the previous one but now it is related to achieving a defined objective. That makes the difference. Within a profession and related to a certain task you will find different methods, sometimes hundreds of them. A method is helpful in implementing the basic methodology. For professionals it is important and often difficult to identify the productive and effective methods. Each method has its own application and quite often it requires study and training to be used. One of the professional skills – part of the methodology – is the competence to identify and select the proper methods for a certain goal.

An instrument

An instrument is a precise specified and prescriptive action to achieve a certain activity or task. The most important difference with a method is the prescriptive and precise character. A method is something to transfer into an action, an instrument is predicting every step within an action. It represents a highly protocolized way of acting.

In reality the three terms partly overlap. We can find a basic methodology for social professionals, as well as for the different professions separately (social work, community work, therapeutic work, social pedagogy work, etc.) within social work. The distinction between methods and instruments is not clear cut.

The methodology of social professionals

In dealing with a methodology bridging the different social professionals, we are actually discussing a 'meta-methodology', a common architectural design in social work. I have tried to construct such a methodology for discussion and elaboration. The main question is whether it is useful and applicable.

Basically, in books about methodologies and methods three main stages can be distinguished:

1   Preparation or planning: looking, listening, understanding, analysing, reflecting, constructing, designing, testing, planning the activities.
2   Action: carrying out the project, the research, the intervention, the activity.
3   Conclusion: evaluation, accounting for, implementation.

Each person is going through this process regularly. Going on holiday needs preparation (where to go, what to take with us, with whom, what activities) and evaluation (never going again to this place and remembering to take swimming costumes next time). Many of us, perhaps, have a holiday checklist, a methodology for the professional tourist.

Planning

Orientation

Something starts with an idea, a brainwave, an identified problem, a request or an assignment. The initiative comes from the authorities, the management, the client, the residents, colleagues or from the professional. Whatever, there is a beginning and now the process starts. The first question is to be certain about the origin of the idea and what the initiators are really wanting. Quite often, the whole process goes wrong already in this very first stage as the real need, the problem or assignment has not been clearly identified. Too quickly, professionals start with finding solutions instead of analysing the need, problem, assignment a little closer. Understanding the context is one of the essentials in good social work. The next step is investigation. What do we know about the person, the situation? What has already been done? Are there experiences and practices to learn from? Who is the target group and are those people waiting for an action? Here, quite often we find too optimistic interpretations. Social workers are often not wanted, seen as threatening or poking their noses in what is not their business.

You need sensitivity for assessing the urgency, the responsiveness, the opportunities, the risks, the different perspectives from different actors. If needed, you study theories (psychological, sociological, juridical and social policy) and look for good practices. The intensity of those investigating steps depends of course on the complexity, the budget, the need, the time available.

Definition

The first step is to define as precisely as possible the problem, or the assignment, or the idea, the request, and to check if this is in line with the important actors, like the user, the financier and the manager. The next step is to identify and formulate the objectives, the conditions (organizational, financial, staffing, etc.), and to identify appropriate methods. In complex cases we need not only objectives and methods but a comprehensive overall strategy as well. Regarding objectives, it is often useful to distinguish different levels of objectives. The first level is to connect the objective to an overall programme or plan, for example, the community programme or the youth care intervention programme or the personal treatment plan. The second level is to define as precisely as possible the goals of this specific intervention, project, activity or research. This intervention-related objective should be clear, achievable and explicit in its intended and presumed outcomes. A third level is the sub-goals or the objectives per activity or action within a project or plan.

Design

This is the third step in the planning or preparation phase. It is the most creative and constructive time within this first stage. Now a concrete plan or strategy has to be developed. What are we where and when, for whom and with whom, and how? What are we going to do and why? We are writing a kind of play script and after drafting the plan we reflect on and discuss the possible outcomes, the risks and opportunities. It is important to imagine how the participant(s) will perceive the actions and how they will react. The better the design is, the better and more confident you can carry out the task. However, it is all about working with people and therefore unpredictable elements are always in it and redesigning is often necessary. At this stage we have to select proper methods but the list of methods and instruments in social work is endless. The number of different professions, different settings and different perspectives and even opinions creates a pile of methods. Even for very similar interventions many different methods exist, each of them claiming to be important and (probably) effective. A social professional cannot oversee, let alone learn and apply all those methods. Therefore, one of the essential things in the methodology is to identify, compare and select the proper methods, and it asks for methods-searching and methods-assessing competences. In this selective process the first question is about the context and objectives. Does the method fits in this context, in those objectives? The second question is about the complexity in application. Is this method easy to adapt and to transfer to our planned action or intervention? The third question is about the quality of the action, in particular its effects and side-effects. Another question asks for the personal fit. Does this method suit me?

Warning

We need to include and connect as much as possible with the users (clients, residents, target group) in defining the problems and to test the design together with users as well.

Table 4.1 Investigating and defining the starting position (problem, request, idea)

	Orientation	investigating the context investigating existing experiences and practices looking into theories
Preparation	Definition	objectives (overall, specific)
	Design	what, where, when, for whom, with whom, how, why selection of methods drafting a plan drafting a working structure

Action

Action means carrying out the plan, doing the job. As a matter of fact, this stage is less systematized than the other two. This is mainly due to the fact that actions differ highly from each other. In other words the difference in carrying out a cultural event or an intervention in a multi-problem family is hard to compare. Carrying out actions is about personal qualities, the professional attitude and the application of methods and instruments. The professional should have the qualities and knowledge to apply methods and to interact with users. The interactive quality or connecting competence are quite basic and ask sometimes for flexibility and at other times for steadfastness. At the same time, in carrying out actions reflection and adjustment are needed. You cannot continue carrying out a plan if the circumstances are changing or nothing works out as planned. Therefore, the basic methodology of a social professional is flexibility in itself and you can go back to an earlier stage if necessary.

	Do	what is in the plan and design apply the methods properly use the instruments be focused
Action	Reflect	be aware of what is happening reflect and rethink
	Adjust	the method if needed the attitude if needed the strategy, plan and design if needed

Conclusion

Concluding an intervention or action is the third stage. It starts with the evaluation: what has been done, how have we done it, what we consider to be the strong and weak points in the planning and design and in the action itself, in the conditional things (time, budget, structure, buildings, etc.) and working together. Did we include the participants properly in the planning and actions? This evaluation can be done by the professionals but it is much better to include users and managers as well. Next we should try to identify the outcomes: results and effects. Results are the things we have done, such as the number of participants, or the number of sessions, the products. Effects or outcomes refer to what has been improved, or to what extent the objectives have been met. To interview users and to measure, for example, satisfaction is a first step. A second one is to investigate if there are sustainable effects, which is very costly to do but is essential in the long run for the motivation of professionals and legitimacy.

Apart from evaluation, we distinguish accountability. We are accountable to our users, managers and financiers. It takes place orally and is often written as well. It is useful to discuss with financiers, managers and clients what they expect, what they will keep you accountable for before starting the action. Accounting for your work and actions has become more important in the last few years. The new management approach expects from all kind of professionals an adequate insight and transparency in what has been done, for what reason and with what results. There is nothing wrong with that. The question is, what we are accounting for and in what way, and if it is reasonable. But again, do not forget the users. This is even more important than satisfying the management. You must inform your users about the process, the products and effects.

The third stage in concluding the action is to take care of the implementation and guarantee a certain sustainability of the process and outcomes. Most of the social activities are aiming to improve something or someone in the long run. Actually, quite often treatments, actions and innovations have an effect in the short run. However, in the long run, the effects disappear. Social work is not just about pleasing people. It is changing behaviour, relationships, situations and, in concluding an action or intervention, social professionals have a responsibility to do all they can to support sustainability.

	Evaluation	process outcomes (products, results, effects) what has been done, why and how effective
Conclusion	Accounting for	the management and financier the user, participant, client the process and the outcomes
	Implementation	sustainability creating supporting conditions

Co-operation and embedment

In the basics of social profession methodology co-operation and embedment are core issues. Co-operation implies that social professionals do not work in a vacuum, but are always active in a field with different actors and different perspectives. 'Social' means indeed working together. Social professionals are most effective in their work if they include users, residents, other professionals and managers and authorities in their actions. They have to connect to the social fabric, the social infrastructure and the social systems. However, many social professionals have the feeling that they are doing their projects and activities in isolation, missing support from their managers and colleagues. The modern way of project and product orientation strengthens this feeling of standing alone (Waal 2007). On the other hand, citizens complain about social professionals not understanding them, not listening properly and to 'professionalize' their problems and activities (Lipsky 1980). In one of my own researches, social professionals were regarded as passers-by, not as someone who is 'belonging to' or 'working for' your community (Maas *et al.* 2008). In this respect of working together on social problems, there is much to be improved, and an interactive way of dealing with problems in social work should become even more the very basis of the methodology.

'Embedment' refers to the strategic and practical connection from an action or intervention to overall plans, programmes and treatment. Piecemealing social interventions has been analysed very often (Castells 1999). Piecemeal programming means that actions are isolated and therefore are not effective. In youth care it is not enough to treat a person in an isolated room. It is necessary to involve the family, the informal network, the school. In community work, overall plans to improve the neighbourhood integrating different sectors is the best way to act. Within those plans and strategies social work is a partner and should connect properly to this framework.

Finally, working together is a difficult job, particularly in the open and unpredictable context of social work. The social domain is for everybody and social professionals should position themselves in the social fabric, respecting users and citizens and residents. It often creates confusion about positions, roles and qualities in relation to citizens and policy makers, professionals from neighbouring sectors and the local authorities.

Three powers in social processes

At the end of the basics in the (meta) methodology of social work I will point out the essence of being reflective and transparent in who has the power at which stage of the social process. The essential stages are the definition of the problem, the decision taking and the implementation.

Power of definition

In citizenship-based social work the fundamental effort is to give citizens back the power of defining the problems, the demands and the contexts. In social policy making and social work processes there is a persistent mechanism to investigate, to interview the user(s) involved and then to define the social problems in the offices of the local authorities and in the offices of the institutions or in the office of the social professional. This definition – created outside the context and reach of the user – is leading the intervention. It is essential to give the power of definition of what are the problems in the community, in the family, in the personal life back to the citizen. If citizens need help, front line professionals – not passer-by professionals – co-operate in this defining process. In the neighbourhoods the experts are the residents and front line professionals who are recognized by the neighbourhood and who are familiar with the neighbourhood. Within families, nearby social professionals work together to come to the definition of what is going on and what should be done. This starting point capsizes the whole social policy and social work system because the managers, the specialists and the policy makers are steered from the defining power of the users and steered by the needs starting from the local context. Be aware that this pledge is not about a simple consumer–producer relationship or a demand-and-supply connection. It is about a thorough process of investigating a context by the context, as needed together with front line professionals! From there, integrated approaches bringing together different expertise and experts and bringing together different logics and institutional powers should start.

Power of decision

In case professional expertise is needed – and agreed – decisions should be taken about budgeting, about staffing (who), about a plan and about conditions. The power of decision is in the hands of the financiers. This is not in the power of the user. Of course the social problem definition should be the basis for the plan and budget and of course the user should be consulted, but the decision is unmistakabley a decision of the agency in charge of budgeting and staffing.

Power of implementation

Maybe the most complicated and controversial question in the social domain is the responsibility for the implementation of the treatment, the intervention or action. From social interventions it is argued and supported by research that approximality 40 per cent of the success of a treatment is due to the user (Yperen 2004, Duncan 2006). Safety, health, education depend greatly on the commitment and interest of the citizen(s). The vitality of a community depends on the quality of civil society. Care and welfare aims cannot be fulfilled without the users. Activating citizenship is essentially connected to this convincing assumption. However, recognizing the citizenship value in solving social problems does not imply the idea that professionals are making citizens dependent or that social professionals are not needed at all. On the contrary, in the highly developed activating welfare state and in our socio-cultural era, supportive interventions for the most vulnerable citizens and communities are very much needed and in line with a social Europe. Implementation of social support, social interventions and social strategies ask for a shared power from citizens, professionals and policy makers.

Competences[2]

In current social work, competences are dominant in expressing the qualities and capabilities social workers need. We shall go into a little more detail on this issue of competences because it is defining the profession and education of social workers to an increasing extent. Competences are helpful for professionals to assess their own qualities. To what extent are those competences already realized and can be improved? This is a challenging question for each professional. It is one means of a reflective investigation of personal abilities. A second impact of competences is their consequences for employers and working conditions. For employers of professional social services, it is important to have a fit between the professionality needed and the workforce. Competence schemes are useful to assess the internal quality of the workforce. The most striking impact of competences is in the higher education system itself. Nearly all universities in Europe have moved or are moving towards a competence-based learning.

What competences are

Definition

We can find thousands of definitions of competences. Look at this one. 'A competence is the integration of knowledge, skills, attitude and reflection applied to a specific task in a certain context and contributing to an appropriate performance and result.' The integration, the application in a context, the performance and the result are essential. Competences are helpful for professionals and educators in investigating what is needed for a certain profession. Many universities base their curriculum on competence schemes which implies integrated learning of skills, knowledge, attitude and reflection. Mostly the learning process starts with a concrete problem in a specific context and from there theories, practices and skills are explored.

Competences and knowledge

Social work knowledge and learning used to be based on the recognition and study of different fields or disciplines such as psychology, sociology and pedagogy as the mothers of social work and helpful fields such as law, economics, social policy, anthropology, history, philosophy, ethics, communication and management. Apart from that, communication skills, creative skills, methods and instruments were studied and training was given. Competence learning *and* separately exploring the main fields of knowledge are the best ways to master social work as a profession at undergraduate and Masters degree level.

Levels of competence

It is debatable if competences should have different levels. It can be argued that different levels of professionalism demand different competences. On the other hand we may hope that an experienced worker will have mastered a competence on a higher level than a novice social worker. For that reason we can distinguish a competence for a starting professional and a senior professional. In that sense we can also argue that students are gradually mastering the competence and we can measure progress. So, we have competences on an 'embryo' level. Universities can create profiles for students where some competences should be mastered at a higher level than others, for example, a social work researcher, a social policy profession and a street-level social worker need different profiles. Some competences are more dominant and should be mastered on a higher level in one profile than in another. Criteria for different levels of mastering a competence are complexity, independence, responsibility, risks and transfer as the quality to use the competence in different contexts and the capacity to transfer knowledge and skills to colleagues, students and the organization.

Assessments

To certify professionals and students finding a proper way of assessing their competences is needed. Such an assessment is different from more traditional ways of assessment, mainly based on knowledge testing and the capability to draft reports and write a thesis. The most proper way to assess competences is to combine different methods:

1   performance assessment in simulating situations or in practice;
2   portfolio assessment based on materials, reflections, products from the student;
3   case analysis and problem-solving solutions;
4   self- , peer, client and staff evaluation (360° assessment), asking the different actors to evaluate a competence of the student by scoring lists or more descriptive information.

The next question to ask is who is responsible for the assessment. It is argued that assessment by an independent authority, not the supervisor and teachers of the students, is preferable. Some universities, therefore, have set up independent assessment centres. The consequence could be that assessments are open for everybody who thinks he or she has mastered the competence. A university degree should no longer be a certificate for having completed a curriculum and passed an exam, but for the mastery of a set of competences.

The competences in social work

Competences are based on analysing professional tasks. Each task asks for certain skills and knowledge. To inform and to consult users properly you need skills like listening, observing, explaining and knowledge about law, services, psychology, sociology, etc. In this way all the professional tasks are split up into elements. The next step is to review all those elements and to categorize them into core competences. A helpful scheme is to divide competences into three areas: primary process competences, managerial competences and the professional competences. The problem is that an internationally agreed categorization of competences is missing. Competences are dependent on the definition of social work, the number of social professions and their profile in a certain country. Competences are in this sense contextual and need to be re-invented in different countries, different regions and different schools and universities. As a matter of fact it is up to the employers and employees (including the government(s) and local authorities) to decide about the competences and it is up to the schools and universities to implement competences into the curriculum.

Primary process competences

Primary process competences are directly connected to the practice of social work. It is about performing a proper execution of the activities as a social worker in meeting the users or clients or participants or consumers or whatever.

THE COMPETENCE TO COMMUNICATE PROPERLY WITH ALL KIND OF USERS

Social professionals are supposed to have the quality to connect to and communicate from very different groups of users, for example, children, people with learning difficulties, people with mental health problems, homeless people and people from different ethnic backgrounds. The competence of communication refers not only to communicating skills but to communicating skills in highly different contexts as well. Clients of social services quite often complain about not being understood, not being treated respectfully or getting the wrong support. To communicate properly is complicated and time consuming. Important skills are listening, observing, analysing, interpretation, explaining, reflecting, searching for information, coming to an agreement. You need knowledge about law, social services, social rights, cultural backgrounds, psychology, sociology, information technology and methods of communication and interpretation.

THE COMPETENCE TO ASSESS CONTEXTS, PEOPLE, NEEDS AND ACTIONS

Quite often social workers have to analyse the strong and weak points on the individual level, network level or even neighbourhood or district level. Dossiers, conversations, questionnaires, diagnostic instruments are resources to get the information from. In certain areas (youth care, long term care) protocols and evidence-based instruments are prescribed. Mostly, however, social workers have to make their own estimation of what is going on and what is needed and what to do. In more complicated cases the social worker tries to get information from different areas such as personal history, networks, school, housing, income, behaviour, relationships, personal functioning and disorders. The resources and hindering factors should be analysed as well. What can we expect from a person, a network, a neighbourhood to be able to cope with and what not, and how can we strengthen the personal quality of coping and how are we able to change things in the environment (networks, school, employer) to make it more supportive for the person involved?

THE COMPETENCE TO PLAN A SOCIAL WORK PROCESS

Social professionals are supposed to take responsibility for carrying out social work activities. A main element in this process is to plan a social service, an activity, an innovation and an intervention properly. An important quality is to connect a project or activity to the needs of the person(s) involved and to the strategy, tasks and procedures of the agency and the financier. Another aspect of planning is to be precise in planning, administration of budgets and time and in reporting.

THE COMPETENCE TO CARRY OUT THE PLANNED PROCESS

The most important competence is to carry out the planned process or service. It is good to relate this competence to what we called the core tasks of social work (pp. 71–2), translated into seven (sub)competences:

1   The competence *to inform, consult and refer people properly*. Asking for knowledge in fields such as law, mapping the domain, communication skills and consulting techniques.
2   The competence *to activate people*. Here methods in bringing people back to work, school, family, social life are to be applied.
3   The competence *to endorse social cohesion*. This competence is much emphasized in modern Europe because of the perceived tensions in societies and communities. The way to do it, to give the competence hands and feet, is still partly lacking.
4   The competence *to develop (or train) social competences*. This is the educating tradition in social work about training people in social skills and social behaviour. It is mostly a core task in youth work, youth care and rehabilitation.
5   The competence *to manage care*. This is particularly needed in social care but in social work with multi-problem families as well. It is taking care of co-ordination and co-operation in solving multidimensional problems. A specific approach in care management is 'support' as a (semi) permanent process of being present and committed to the person to take care of and to support the person in getting the things done.
6   The competence *to intervene*, to act directly and improve a situation by different interventions such as mediation, crisis intervention, taking a child out of the family, all kind of therapies.
7   The competence *to supervise and control*. This often neglected competence demands social professions who are able to interfere, to take decisions and actions that are felt as enforcing and are not wanted by the user. Supervising

and controlling asks for assessing critical situations and monitoring users' context carefully.

Those seven (sub)competences in carrying out the planned process ask for different knowledge and skills. At the same time they are part of the overall competence of social workers to provide support or help to their users. Included in these competences is the capability to select and apply existing methods, to adjust them and, if needed, to innovate new approaches. These core tasks of the social professional are always related to specific settings, such as target group, place, specific objectives and expressed needs or demands.

THE COMPETENCE TO CO-OPERATE

Here we are discussing the quality of working together with different people on the same case or in the same contexts. You should have the capability to co-operate with other professionals, volunteers, informal carers and people in networks of your user. In particular, networking has attracted much attention in the last few years. In support and intervention the role of nearby people is seen as very relevant to improving the problems and position of the person in need. Social work is mainly contextual work, working in the field where individuals, networks, systems (school, labour market, health, justice) and community or society are interactive creating patterns, cultures and behaviour.

Managerial competences

Managerial competences are those connected to employees and professionals within an organization, maybe a social service in the public sector or a NGO or private enterprise.

THE COMPETENCE TO ADAPT TO AN ORGANIZATION

Social workers are mostly employed by an organization. The professional position depends on the mission, tasks and profile of this agency. Social professionals are often deeply engaged in the process of supporting people and have hardly any interest in the organization they work for. In their ideas an organization is something that pays salaries, something you work in but not for. However, modern social services are aiming to be professional organizations, which imply that they have their own professionalism. It is more than hosting professionals. A social professional should adapt to the mission, tasks, rules and strategy of his or her agency and contribute to the development of the agency as well. Adapting in this respect is a mutual process aiming at improving the quality of the organization as such and its professionals as well. The competence has to do with qualities like being a good colleague, to accept and communicate with your manager, to represent your organization and to network in your organization.

Social professionals, in particular those educated to Masters level, should have the basic competence to manage a team or department. To be a good manager you need to have different capabilities. First, you have to run your unit properly in respect of financing, controlling and planning. Second, you need leadership skills to direct your people, to endorse them, to evaluate their capacities and to improve their competences and output. Third, you should be able to develop strategic policies for the future direction of your unit, to contribute to the strategy of your organization and to implement strategies and innovations. Fourth, you need to be acquainted with quality management, the regular process of analysing, evaluating and improving your unit. Human resource management, some accounting experiences like budgeting and basic financial administration and strategic thinking are essential for a manager.

THE COMPETENCE TO DEVELOP AND IMPLEMENT SOCIAL POLICIES

A social worker is not a stand-alone professional with a fully independent role in society, comparable with general practitioners. Social professionals are part of social politics and are seen as rather instrumental. They should co-operate in activating people, in supporting vulnerable people, in protecting people and sometimes protecting society and so on. Social politics are always changing, as discussed extensively. A social professional is not doing good – oh yes, she or he often does but that is not why she or he is paid – but helping society to meet its objectives, such as participation, welfare and caring for certain kinds of people. Social workers have a lot of practical knowledge of people's lives and how systems are working and affecting the vulnerable people in society. In that respect they should contribute to improve and develop social policies. Their knowledge and expertise in this respect is needed. On the other hand, social policy makers draft plans, lay down intentions and make direction. They need social professionals to make it work. Social professionals have the quality to transfer social policy into effective practice.

Professional competences

Professional competences imply the capability to stand for your profession, your professional expertise and for employability, planning your own career, horizontally and vertically.

TO PLAN YOUR OWN PERSONAL CAREER

This is the competence related to employability. Employability means the capability to be active and attractive in the labour market by lifelong learning, mobilization, developing new competences and deepening existing competences. Social professionals should safeguard and deepen their reflection on their own acting and thinking and on what is happening in the context they work in and for. It is about keeping the interest in personal development, the curiosity in the world around you, the commitment to the profession you work in. On the one hand the basic attitude of a professional is to broaden his or her knowledge (new areas in knowledge and practice) and to deepen it (to specialize), and on the other hand to change his or her position horizontally (another field of service) and/or vertically (higher position). It is all about employability, the capacity to keep in line with developments in the profession and labour market and to adapt to new demands.

TO PROFILE AND PRESENT YOURSELF AND YOUR PROFESSION

Social workers are by nature hardly focused on profiling their own quality and importance or representing their profession and branch. The basic attitude is to help and support other people. Quite often social professionals are lacking a clear concept and overview of their profession, their professional domain and the existing body of knowledge. They are also unclear about relating their own profession and position to other social professions and related professions (in health, education, law). They often do not have international and academic orientations and connections. Besides a lack of awareness and pride to be a social worker they should be able to explain the profession, its importance and contribution to society and the evidence of its interventions, clearly and convincingly.

TO INNOVATE PRACTICES AND METHODS

Here we discuss whether this competence belongs to the professional competences or primary process competences. It can be regarded as professional because it does not refer in the first place to the capability to innovate in daily practice but to a permanent or immanent capability of a social professional to be innovative in the primary process, in the managerial competences and in the social professional's own professional competences. This competence emphasizes that modern social professionals are not carrying out tasks alone or in the first place but that an important role is to improve and change practice.

Competence-based learning

Competence-based learning asks for a certain adjustment of the curriculum.

1   It should be verified if the current curriculum in principle meets the competences. There are certainly gaps, overlaps or redundant pieces in the curriculum.
2   Competence learning asks for a different learning concept, based more on learning from problem-solving cases, practice or practice simulation, and additionally lectures in related areas of knowledge (disciplines, theories, research), skills training (for example, communication, counselling) and coaching (reflection, critical support, guidance).

3   Competence learning asks for competence-based assessments, such as performance assessment, portfolio assessment, self- , peer and staff assessments and evidence from theoretical, reflective and research products (theses, essays, tests, researches).

The social professional

By way of a summary we define the citizenship-based social professional. This professional is fully aware of living and working in a permanent transforming context. Shifts in social policy and the diversity of residents are highly relevant for professionals. The first perspective is on activation and participation. It is expected that these professionals that create their own professional career path profile, based on affinities, competences, experiences and deliberate choices. The profile can be more directed towards front line generalist work, or entrepreneurship and innovation or on being a specialist in a certain field or method. The roots can be grounded more in social pedagogy, social work, community work, social care, therapeutic work or community art work. The professional connects theories, practices and policies. The body of knowledge is based on the professional practice, social work theories and neighbouring scientific fields and coloured by citizenship-based social work. The professional is competent in bridging, in activation, in understanding, research and planning actions, in caring, consulting, endorsing, intervening and training. The social professional has a strong awareness of the role, position and responsibility in relation to local social policy, the service provider and the citizen (as partner, employer, consumer or client) and accounts for the work done for the different stakeholders, to start with the users.

Discussion and assignment

Discussion

We present four statements, asking you to comment on the statements.

1   Social work stands for a broad domain of different professions. It is important to accept a common body of knowledge as a basis for the different social professions. Social professionals need a convincing and recognizable identity to bind them together. So far, the field is too fragmented.
2   The citizen-based social work definition is preferable to the Montreal definition. Discuss.
3   Students should learn at university to be basically competent in different positions (front line worker, entrepreneur, specialist), in different social professions and in different core tasks.
4   Social professionals are free to choose their own social work theory (approach).

Reflection

It is important to reflect on all the differences regarding social work and to think about your own point of view. Just go through the different sections again and see which root, discourse, core task, theory, position, etc. is most appealing to you. It helps you to profile your own professional career.

Considering the (meta)methodology, do you recognize it as a base for all social professions?

What is your opinion about the last paragraph 'the social professional'; does it appeal to you?

Assignment

Please fill in the three tables below using a 1 to 5 scale (5 = fully mastered, 1 = not). 'Mastered' refers to the extent you think you have mastered this competence, core task or field of knowledge. 'Importance' means how important this competence, task and field of knowledge is for you. 'Thanks to my university' asks how much you feel you have learnt or mastered the competence, core tasks of field of knowledge at your university.

Competences	Mastered	Importance	Thanks to my university
1 To communicate properly			
2 To assess contexts and needs			
3 To do research			
4 To plan a social work process			
5 To carry out the planned process			
6 To co-operate			
7 To adapt to an organization			
8 To manage			
9 To relate to social policies			
10 To plan your personal career			
11 To profile and present your self/your profession			
12 To innovate practices and methods			

Core tasks	Mastered	Importance	Thanks to my university
To inform, to consult			
To activate			
To endorse social cohesion			
To develop social competences			
To manage care			
To intervene			
To supervise and control			

Fields of knowledge	Mastered	Importance	Thanks to my university
Psychology			
Sociology			
Pedagogy			
Anthopology			
Law			
Social policy			
Social work theories			
Social work methodology			
Social work methods and instruments			
Social work practice			
Social management			
Communication, public relations			

5 Community policy and community work

Introduction

In eighteenth-century London, it became popular to 'transport' criminals to Australia and other parts of the world. The remarkable thing was that criminality rates were hardly decreasing in London and the criminality rates in Australia were quite low (Hughes 1987). It seems to be that expelling criminals does not solve the problem of criminality. In the ghettos of the modern US about 90 per cent of African-American boys are accused of (supposed) criminal behaviour (Wacquant 1999). This is not due to a genetic disorder but most likely due to the fact that they grow up in places where you can hardly escape being involved in criminality. Disturbed communities provoke disturbed behaviour and disturbed relationships. Cultural patterns do have an impact on the mind or habitus of people (Bourdieu 1984). Individuals interact with other individuals and systems and the entirety of interactions or patterns can be supportive or disturbing for those individuals.

Community-based social policy

Social work has always had three perspectives on social action. The first looks at individuals and their networks. The second starts with a certain category or group: children, marginalized youth, the elderly, ethnic minorities, the disabled, etc. The third perspective is on a certain territory: a neighbourhood, a community, a village. In this chapter we deal with local social policy aiming at strengthening local communities, such as neighbourhoods and districts.

A short history of the (local) community concept

The great Greek philosophers, Socrates, Plato, and Aristotle, were convinced that the local community (polis) was a basic condition for life. Living together was presumption for individual life. In former times people were born, lived and died in the same community. The local community created a pattern for life, a shared and recognized world and shared values. At least that was the principle. In fact, wars, famine, contagious diseases caused often mass migrations. Until today, a community is characterized by relationships (networks), recognition, shared values and a feeling of belonging and trust (Etzioni 1993, 1998 Putnam 2000,). The Pilgrim Fathers, one of the very first groups of settlers in the US, were very successful in economic production. One of the supposed reasons for their success was the fact that the first thing they did after settling was to build together a community centre for religion, meetings, actions, policy making, culture (Keller 2003). The idea that a community does things together was symbolized and applied in this community centre and this community feeling empowered them to take risks, to be entrepreneurs and to create a culture of mutual trust. For the Greek philosophers the community is about morality, a political order steered by a well educated elite (Plato). It refers to the virtues of the leading people and their belief in the community, the polis. In the Roman empire the state, the empire and its emperor were the centre of power. Laws, rules and discipline were the binding forces for communities (Cato). The Christian religion, which diffused very quickly in the late Roman period, focused on the overarching power as well. The Civitas Dei (Augustine) was based on a common God, on a common belief and submission to the Church represented in and by the Pope. The local community was held together by its religion, the Church and the nobility. In the seventeenth and eighteenth centuries, a new way of thinking introduces rationalism and utility as fundamentals for communities. What binds communities together is the common good, the common interest (John Stuart Mill, Thomas Hobbes, Aquinus). Later, Rousseau nuanced this idea in his theory of the social contract. However, in all these different ideas about the binding force of society, philosophers perceived the local community as fundamental to human life. In the eighteenth and nineteenth centuries mobility and rational knowledge increased quickly and the traditional binding forces in the local community gradually lost their integrating capacity. Therefore, the idea of democracy – having its roots in Greek and Roman times, and existing thousands of years ago in states of India as well – became dominant in the nineteenth century in the Western world, having its Western European predecessors in, for example, the English Parliament (1265). The French Revolution shook up the traditional 'stable' society, built on a fixed hierarchical structure and minimum mobility for most people into a democratic way of organizing societies and communities. After the French Revolution philosophers were puzzled again by what holds communities together in this modern society. Hierarchy, stability and religion were losing their binding power. In simple terms, the founders of sociology found different answers, as we saw in Chapter 2 with Weber focusing on the bureaucracy and the state, Marx on his belief in the classless society and solidarity as the binding power, and Durkheim on the society as a productive community where each individual has their role and place, bound together by the fact that everybody contributes to the productive society. Labour was the binding force and industries should be co-operative communities that hold people together (Durkheim 1986). We can argue that none of the three founders of sociology forecasted correctly. The welfare state seems to maintain itself and to bind people by providing affluence, freedom and a certain level of equality. However, at the end of the twentieth century the interest in the integrative power of the state, the society and the local communities came prominently back on the social agenda. Concepts like social cohesion, diversity, participation and integration express the feeling that societies are losing their integrative power for different reasons (see also Chapter 2).

1   The increasing mobility of people created problems and conflicts in many societies. A growing diversity needed new answers to the integrative power of society and communities.
2   Globalization put pressure on societies to decrease public expenditure, calling for a more active, and risk-taking civil society.
3   The welfare state (or communist state) is changing into a workfare state or an activating welfare state.
4   In the poor districts of big cities and in many rural communities social structures eroded, and anonymity became threatening.
5   Criminality and feelings of insecurity increased.
6   In a number of welfare states populism and (extreme) right-wing political parties were very successful on issues like safety, anti-multiculturalism and liveable environments. Much was about a desire for a safe and secure world, for communities to feel home again.

The modern welfare state focused on a delivering state and the citizen as an individual person, protected by democratic and social rights. There was not much room for communities as basic entities for an integrative power in this concept. Freedom, affluence and rights dominated the discourse. Fraternity was often felt as belonging to religion and old-fashioned traditions and exclusively restricted to private life and personal responsibility. Recently, communities, in particular the local community, seem to be the dominant answer to the recognition that human relationships and decent social behaviour are necessary assets for a cohesive society.

Re-inventing the local community

We will analyse the revival of the local community in a little more detail by summing up a number of social policies aiming at strengthening communities.

Contextual approaches and localization

We discussed an important drive back to the communities in Chapter 2. Socio-economic dominance in social policy became more balanced by socio-cultural issues. Social cultural problems about human conflicts, relationships, inappropriate individual behaviour are mostly experienced in one's own municipality, in the neighbourhood and on the street. To tackle negative social feelings and to intervene in social conflicts, local action seems the most effective. Social cultural policy is highly contextual and local. In many nations, decentralization of social policy to the local policy has been implemented or is planned. The responsibility for the citizens' wellbeing and behaviour is most visible in the community and is often seen as a shared responsibility by the local authorities, the citizen(s), civil society and the services.

Community care

Community care got its modern impact on social work in the Barclay Report in 1982, produced under a conservative government with Margaret Thatcher as Prime Minister (NISW 1982). The Barclay Report stated that community care involving family, friends and neighbourhoods is the way to organize care. It implied de-institutionalization, local responsibility and strengthening civil society and informal care. Community care could keep care affordable and could ensure sufficient hands to care. This idea spread over Europe and is the leading concept in most countries. The focus on providing care at home and by involving family, volunteers and professionals in the right mix is attractive because it appeals to social responsibility, civil society and enables people to live in their own homes and neighbourhoods and of course for economic reasons. Community care created new roles for social workers as being the case or care managers in complicated contexts.

'It takes a village to raise a child'

Hillary Clinton, quoting an old African proverb 'It takes a village to raise a child' (Clinton 1996), expressed a third concept: influencing community thinking. The proverb assumes that educating a child needs a consistent and coherent place to grow up. Family, school, leisure time activities, services and all kind of networks should co-operate in the process of upbringing. Clinton's book and speech stress the fact that upbringing is not merely a task – and sometimes problem – of the family or mother. This kind of perception brought the community back on the youth policy agenda. Similar to the caring community approach, the community approach in the field of educating children appeals to families, friends and neighbours to feel responsible for people around them (Cannan and Warren 1997). The US developed – but implemented in several European countries – a youth preventive programme 'Communities that care' which starts from the same assumption that the neighbourhood is the place to prevent and to intervene when young people are at risk (CTC 2008).

The safe and secure neighbourhood

The idea to intervene in the neighbourhood or at local community level seems also to be fruitful in fighting against criminality. Programmes such as *community policing* have been evaluated as successful (Donovan and Walsh 1989). Community policing aims at co-operation with residents in crime prevention; for example, in programmes like neighbourhood watch. In a more broadened scope, it involves all kinds of actors in the community and aims at agreed plans and co-operation to improve the safety in the community. In its extreme examples, gated or fenced communities are the solutions for the rich or the elderly (Sanchez *et al.* 2005).

Revitalizing neighbourhoods

Local policy makers endorse, strengthen, revitalize and promote safe communities or neighbourhoods (East 2002, Keller 2003, Hardcastle and Powers 2004, Smith 2006). Modern community work is trying to integrate physical (buildings, urban planning and environment), economic and social sectors at neighbourhood or district level (Jacobs 1992, East 2002, Ellison and Pierson 2003). It enhances the attraction of neighbourhoods by improving services, by influencing the composition of the community residents, by improving environmental aspects, safety in the neighbourhood and by endorsing social cohesion, diversity and participation. Housing co-operatives, urban planners and local authorities have a great interest in this aspect of strengthening communities because attractive neighbourhoods increase the prices of houses and the neighbourhoods become more attractive for economic activities.

Integration and diversity

There is a massive debate on multiculturalism, diversity and integration, mainly referring to marginal ethnic groups (Banks and Banks 1989, Taylor 1992, Bauböck and Rundell 1998, Ayaan 2006). Most experts pledge for diversity or multiculturalism. Again, the neighbourhoods are seen as an important approach for those integration policies. Many outbursts and riots in the field of ethnic conflicts are in certain areas in the big cities (*banlieues*) and have to be dealt with by investing in those communities. Many local social policy documents focus highly on integration in the community by education, collaborative activities, sports, culture and intervention strategies.

De-institutionalization

De-institutionalization aims at keeping people in their own families and communities. In most countries people with serious disorders, mental health, learning, psychiatric, physical or with social-psychological problems were placed in institutions that took care of them. For some decades the trend was reversed. The modern idea is to care for people at home because institutions institutionalize people and isolate them from society. For that reason, the institutions have transformed themselves into a number of small units spread over the surrounding cities and villages. De-institutionalization fits in with the rediscovery of the local community as the place to be and the place to be cared for.

Participation and civil society

Since Putnam (1993, 2000) scientists and policy makers are fully aware that participation and involvement of civil society is one of the most important resources for the economic and social success of local communities (or regions or countries). Strong communities create and strengthen financial, human and social capital. Putnam demonstrates, albeit contested, that active citizens' involvement in the political arena and in the civil society area is one of the most convincing indicators for wellbeing, welfare and feelings of security. In Putnam's thinking, policy makers should aim at improving residents' participation and involvement in communities.

Along this kind of reasoning in different perspectives, the community is the place to act. Devolution, decentralization and de-institutionalization focus on giving space to communities and civil society 'to take their responsibility'. All actions together aggravate the tasks for communities at the same time. For communities it is demanding to fulfil all these expectations and host so many different (target) groups and care-demanding individuals. And we should not forget that territorial communities are only one of the many communities citizens participate in, from virtual communities, to the workplace, the sporting club, the city, and the family.

The concept of community

Community as concept has been defined from many different angles and there is no internationally agreed definition. It is maybe better to look at the elements found in community definitions. Social bonds, social interaction, connection, recognition, cohesion, common actions, shared values, shared feelings, feelings of belonging are often cited (Keller 2003). Most of those words refer to relationships between certain numbers of people. Those numbers can differ from just a handful to millions of people. In this reader, we restrict the community to a 'physical' one, to a certain definable territory. The connection between community and a certain territory is often made (Keller 2003). The next restriction is that in the community work perspective we always speak about a recognizable dimension, somewhere between 50 and 5,000. A minimal description could be: 'a local community is a small-scale territory where people live.' In this minimal definition, the only things that count are territory and people living in that territory, the so-called 'geographic community' (Regan 2007: 1). Such a community can be an object for policy making, for research, for administration. However, words like 'community work', 'community care' and 'community development' connect to connotations that are more normative. Apparently, we expect something from the community. A more extended description therefore could be: 'a local community is a small-scale territory where people live and interact based on a feeling of belonging and trust.' This expresses 'the community of interest' (Regan 2007: 1). In the minimal definition community research and policy making is restricted to a formal framework: this is the area, those are the people to research or to administrate. In the community of interest policy making and community work are aiming to support community life, social cohesion and social competences. One step further is this one:

> Community work is that portion of activity focused on bringing about social change with a set of working principles, namely; that the process is collective,

participative; is social justice and equality focused; and employs a methodology which is empowering and liberating to individual participants and the
community.

(Chanan 1997)

This definition is not exactly about community but about community work,
but the interesting point is that a specific ideal community has been defined
based on social justice, equality and even liberation. The idea behind adding
those last words is the presumption that strong communities as such are not by
definition positive and inclusive. Communities can be harsh in discriminating
and excluding some members of the community. Therefore, values like social
justice should be added to the idea of the ideal community. The core idea is the
community based on commitment and mutual reciprocity, favoured by Etzioni
(1993) and contested by Bauman (2001). We describe this as 'the idealistic
community'.

I will focus on the second definition, the community as a small-scale territory
where people live and interact based on a feeling of belonging and trust. The
community-based policy aims to foster interaction and participation, and feelings
of security, recognition and mutual sense of responsibility and responsive attitude
to create feelings of belonging and trust. A good neighbourhood to live in is a place
to feel safe, to have good neighbours, to know most people, and to greet them.
Some of them may become friends. People trust each other and the services. It is
a place to feel good and relaxed. It is not asking for a strong community feeling or
great efforts to organize the community. It is more about weak ties and casual
encounters with neighbours (Jacobs 1992, Putnam 2000, Keller 2003). Starting
from this concept of community, interaction and participation should be promoted
and concrete actions to improve mutual connections and informal meetings should
be endorsed. Establishing safety in a neighbourhood is another important aspect
regarding our definition and to implement. Trust is the most difficult one to transfer
into political objectives, however essential. If people do not trust their neighbours,
the street-level professionals (Lipsky 1980) and community, they will leave the
community or at least withdraw from the community as much as possible. Trust is
interdependent with connotations such as recognition, interaction, participation
and a responsive attitude.

Community as habitat

We often conceptualize communities as groups of people who interact. The
emphasis is on people and mutual connections. This interactive process creates
to a certain point a constructed reality that has an impact on its own human
behaviour and human dispositions (Bourdieu and Passeron 1970, Bourdieu 1984).
And even more, it is not only about relationships and patterns among people; it is
as well about interaction between human beings and the physical world: the streets,
the buildings, the parks and the environment. It makes a difference if people grow
up in a small remote village or in the heart of a metropolis. In community policy,

practice and research we should take this interaction between 'habitat' and 'habitus' into account. Habitat stands for a sustainable environment, dependent on the quality of its consistent parts and interactions. Animals can live in a habitat if it is fulfilling the conditions needed. And like animals, human beings need an environment that fits with them. The 'habitat' quality has its impact on the residents (Jacobs 1992). Local communities represent financial capital, social capital and human capital. A community in decline effects a loss in financial, learning and human capital. Therefore, there should be a great interest in the quality of a community to sustain and to develop.

Zones

In community policy and community work, we perceive different zones. A zone is a recognizable field comprising economic, physical and social elements related to a common social assignment. A zone is characterized by the alignment and co-operation between different sectors and services. Social work is part of a chain policy and chain execution of social objectives. Looking at social work we can roughly divide a community into three areas where services are provided and social professionals are employed.

1   The local social education zone. In social education, the focus is on social development, in particular the education of children and young people. It starts with providing services, such as child care, youth centres, information and consultancy for young people and families and school-related social work activities and services. A next layer comprises the more intervention-based services in youth care (mental health, child protection) which are mostly accessible by referrals from professionals and/or accessed by independent agencies. A third layer is based on a more community-based approach. It aims at the whole educational environment, including family, school, leisure time facilities, youth care and the neighbourhood and street level (Bronfenbrenner 1979, 1986, Tolan *et al.* 1995). A fourth layer is to focus on the physical environment, such as streets, houses, playgrounds, parks, public space and traffic.

2   The social care zone. In this zone, the main target group are people in need of long term care. The international trend is to focus on care support enabling elderly, disabled people and people with mental health problems (socio-psychological) to stay in their own home and neighbourhood (Cameron and Moss 2007). This approach asks for a coherent system from home care, to activation, health, and an accessible environment and lifelong sustainable houses and community care as citizen-based supportive systems (Wilken and Hollander 2005). The shift to home-based care support raised new managerial problems because sometimes the support and care for a certain person is very demanding and complex. In this respect a social care profession to manage care, to strengthen networks and to give support is essential and closer to social work than the more caring and nursing professions.

3   The zone of the attractive, safe and secure community. A third zone in social work is to endorse and to promote safe communities and to strengthen and revitalize neighbourhoods (Jacobs 1980, Keller 2003, Hardcastle and Powers 2004). Modern community work is trying to integrate physical (buildings, urban planning and environment), economic and social sectors at neighbourhood or district level. It enhances the 'amenity' (its attraction) of neighbourhoods by improving services, by influencing the composition of community residents, by improving the environmental aspects, safety in the neighbourhood and by endorsing social cohesion, diversity, integration and participation (Ewijk 2009).

For social professionals it is quite important to be aware of the different branches of social work and social professions. It has a great impact on profiling social professionals and in guaranteeing a basic competence level for the different zones.

Community-based social policy

In general, politics and policy-making processes focus on sectors and target groups. Politics refers to different scales, such as global, European Union, national, regional and local. In this respect, a neighbourhood or local community is often not a political entity like a municipality or a state. Neighbourhood or district policies hardly existed, but recently local community policy making has become very popular, as argued above. In urban planning, we have already found overall ideas of building new districts or restructuring neighbourhoods. In social work, ideas about a community approach started in the nineteenth century, for example, community centres (see next section). From the 1950s onwards community (social) policy – often named community development – began to evolve (Thomas 1983, Smith 2006). A characteristic for a community-based social policy is that it aims to improve a community (geographical community) as a habitat. In community-based social policy or community development we distinguish different perspectives. Those partly overlapping perspectives direct concepts, policies and social actions. It is good to recognize the impact of different perspectives.

The grassroots perspective

Derived from social work origins and from social development work in developing countries, one of the strategies to improve life in communities is to empower the marginal people to stand up for their interests. Voicing the excluded is the dominant perspective and social professionals are supposed to support the excluded, sometimes to represent them and to enable them to voice their interests. In the 1960s and 1980s raising social and political awareness became popular (Freire, Giesecke, Deppe). The excluded should become aware that their marginal position is not to blame for a lack of competences but that their position is an outcome of the capitalist system, based on a class society. The grassroots perspective is, for all, a political-based strategy. Community workers are in this perspective, specialized social workers who focus on the grassroots perspective and on empowering the poor. The real grassroots dream is that the poor take full responsibility and get the power for building up their own community,

The educational perspective

At the end of the nineteenth century in London Arnold Toynbee started to encourage educated people to live in marginalized communities and to set up community centres, mainly aimed at educating the excluded in learning and social competences (Jones and Mayo 1974, Thomas 1983). In many poor districts and neighbourhoods, community centres and youth centres were set up to educate the poor. Volunteers and sometimes social workers (social cultural workers or social educators or community workers) established leisure time activities, in particular in the socio-cultural sphere, and all kinds of social activities and a number of educational courses.

Capacity-building perspective

Capacity building expresses the idea that a community should use it own resources and power to develop the community. Local social policy should enable the community by facilitating and empowering strategies to vitalize the community. Professionals are in the background, sometimes providing information, consultation and some services, but the real developing power should come from the community. In the US many communities are organized by volunteers from the community, often driven by a small group of active citizens and often with a recognized 'leader' (Keller 2003).

Participation perspective

The participation perspective is close to the capacity-building process but it emphasizes more the need for participation of all people in the community. Participation refers to all taking part in democratic political processes (voting, debating, decision making) and taking part in volunteering activities (youth work, sports and schools). The idea is that participation as such contributes to a more attractive neighbourhood because active people are meeting each other and developing a more positive attitude (Putnam 2000, Keller 2003). Participation, seen from the perspective of policy makers, creates more support for policy-making processes; it increases the supporting power in a community and prevents expensive professional input.

Planning perspective

The planning perspective refers to a local community as an area for policy making and social planning. In a neighbourhood or district, you need a certain infrastructure (traffic, houses, green areas, schools, social services, shops, etc.) and a comprehensive strategy. What kind of a neighbourhood do people want? Is it for families, for rich people, homogeneous or diverse, for young people or more for elderly people? Should it emphasize privacy or community, flats or independent houses, or a mix? In modern planning approaches it is fashionable to integrate social, economic and physical strategies and to involve the residents in the planning process (Ellison and Pierson 2003).

Managing perspective

In many cities in marginal districts, district managers or account managers are responsible for managing the public and social services in the community. They try to endorse collaboration, to share responsibilities (partnership), and to fine-tune the different activities and services in the community. They promote participation, volunteers and cultural and sporting activities and they liaise with the central administration in the city. This community management requires social managers trained in planning, programming and managing processes.

Communitarian perspective

A community is in the feeling of many people based on shared belonging and a longing for a home. In this communitarian perspective commitment, social involvement and shared values are essential (Etzioni 1993). This approach is often sceptical about the managerial and policy-making perspectives. They analyse those approaches as getting people into the systems instead of starting with the people. The communitarian perspective is more narrative and values based and rather anti-professional.

The complexity of community-based social policy

Conflicting concepts and steering strategies

Community policies are easily conflicting with the central organized policy-making sectors, such as urban planning, security, housing, health, social services or social welfare, education and traffic. In big cities, a programming structure has often been implemented, to integrate different sectors to deal with complex social problems and social assignments on themes like integration, social cohesion, crime prevention, social education or safety. The implementation of a territory oriented community policy adds a third steering principle, competing with sectoral and programming processes. It raises new problems in decision-making power, in defining responsibilities and it causes conflicting interests and difficulties in collaboration. Most municipalities are not very successful at steering this from different angles at the same time (Castells 1999, Keller, 2003, Waal 2007). Another complicating factor is that many locally important actors are not steered at all by the local authorities but are acting in the free market or under responsibility of the state or regional authority. This threefold steering process – sector, programme, territory – creates a new bureaucracy in policy making because of the permanent intensive process of fine-tuning and negotiating between the different scales and different steering processes. However, it is not only about conflicting mechanisms within the sphere of the public sector. Problematic in social policies are also the vague concepts about citizenship, social cohesion, integration, diversity, empowerment, responsibility and so on (Keller 2003, Waal 2007). It creates a certain feeling that we are aiming at the same things but in reality behind those concepts we find completely different feelings and practices.

One of the puzzling problems in community policy is to create a fruitful co-operation between the residents and the professionals from the public sector, from the social services and from the market. It is about a different scale of thinking and acting. Residents identify community life in general with their street, the block where they live, the small-scale neighbourhood. Professionals tend to think on larger scales, such as the district or the city. Time is another discriminating factor. Most residents want it at this moment. Most policy makers and professionals focus on the longer term, among them the urban planners in decades, policy makers in periods of about four years and social workers in weeks or months. Apart from time and scale perceptions, the method of reasoning can be very different. Professionals and policy makers have their own 'logic', not easy for residents to adapt to. Nevertheless, most professionals expect residents to fit into the policy-making processes of the urban planners and social managers.

A last conflicting point is between participative community building as a joint effort from residents, professionals and the public sector and the democratic system. In a democracy, the elected members of the municipality are supposed to take the decisions. In participative processes, active citizens in the neighbourhood have a significant say in the political process. However, seen from the point of view of democratic ideas the principle of just and fair representation is in danger, because participative citizens comprise only a certain number of the residents and mandating decisive power to the neighbourhood is maybe affecting the democratic process.

Different innovation strategies

Community policies are usually aiming at improving the neighbourhood, at development, revitalization and restructuring by innovating approaches and are often driven by rather strong managerial concepts. Quite often those innovation policies are created by additional programmes, projects and budgeting, and by pre-defined outcomes, often expressed in numbers or percentages. In new managerial strategies precise results, concrete projects and activities within a strict time schedule are the instruments to implement the objectives. Innovation is a push from outside to stimulate and seduce actors to do what the managers are aiming for. This approach has been analysed as piecemeal programming (Castells 1999). The projects and programmes are too small, too short in time to bring about a real innovation. Actually, innovation programmes and projects are competing with each other and distracting professionals and residents from their own ideas and activities. The approach is based on discontinuity, temporary impulses, short-term interventions, and mobility and flexibility. Extensive community development programs, such as RAPID (Ireland), New Deal for Communities (UK), are not producing the outcome (Smith 2006, Regan 2007). Suggested positive results are mostly short term improvements in a certain restricted field of activities, thanks to combined and targeted actions. Therefore, a certain shift to more sustainable strategies starting from the actors in the community and based on continuity is necessary. Those strategies focus on long term processes and holistic integrative approaches and mandating the community actors to be responsible for the social development of their own community. The power of innovation is based in the community itself, the residents and front line workers.

Innovation from outside	Innovation from inside
Programming, projects	Organic improvement
Results, effects, outcomes	Processes, gradually
Short term planning	Long term objectives
Managerial driven	Civil society driven
Policy makers responsible	Participative responsibility
Discontinuity	Sustainability

Summary

Summarizing the complicating factors in community-based social policy we have found the following issues:

1 The community is not a formal scale of policy making (no formal authority).
2 There are potential conflicts between sector- , programme- and territory-based policies.
3 Other scales (EU, national, regional) and independent actors are interfering.
4 There are bureaucratic processes in the public sector for harmonizing and fine-tuning.
5 There are different perceptions and cultures between different actors, such as policy makers, managers, professionals and citizens.
6 There is confusion about responsibility, processes of decision making and implementation.
7 There is the problem of unclear concepts, different ideologies and non operational concepts.
8 There is the problem of different scale and time perceptions.
9 There is the problem of reconciling participative processes with democratic principles.
10 Innovation from outside versus innovation from inside.
11 Piecemeal programming versus process and integrative approaches.
12 Aiming at concrete results versus aiming at gradually ongoing development and improvement.
13 Managerial steering versus mandating the community (civil society).

Promising strategies

Transparency and clarity

First, regarding the problematic sides in community-based policies (see above), it is important to create clarity and transparency in different respects, to start with the basic concepts and underlying ideas. An agreement – or recognized and accepted dissensus – on used core concepts, the perceptions, the perspectives and direction is essential. From there, a common understanding of the steering strategy (managerial, mandating, focus on products and results or focus on process, innovation from outside or inside) is necessary. Important in steering and imple-mentation is the perceived and expected role and responsibility from the different parties involved, respecting different cultures, ways of thinking and acting (time and scale). Recognition of a number of impeding realities, such as conflicting sector and integrated approaches, and interfering market and national scale steering processes, is important, and keeping a realistic eye on possibilities and impossi-bilities is needed. For a successful community-based social policy a framework document to define the most important principles, concepts and strategies can be very helpful in getting things done properly.

Local knowledge

Second, it is important to analyse what the problems are in a community. Most community plans lack a reliable analysis and the concept of local knowledge (WRR 2005) has not been really designed, nor implemented. Local knowledge is about the knowledge we need for constructive and effective plans to improve the neighbourhood. Local knowledge is one of the important bases for community-based social work. Local knowledge is often rather fragmented and mostly based on statistics. Local knowledge improves by using the implicit and explicit knowledge of residents and professionals in the community (see below).

Combining strategies

The next question is what kind of strategies and methods are effective when a whole or substantial area in a community is marginalized. In general, the idea is that a range of methods and strategies is needed, striving for coherence and consistency among them. To strengthen and improve living conditions in a deprived community an integrated set of interventions is the best way to go. Let us overview the most important and probably most promising actions (WRR, 2005, VROM 2006, Engberse *et al.*, 2007, Waal 2007).

1   Influencing the composition of the residency. One of the most successful interventions is to change the group of residents, at least successful for this specific neighbourhood. Sometimes it can be effected by restructuring processes. Blocks or streets are demolished and new flats and houses are built, aiming at different target groups, mostly richer and better educated.

By building or renovating houses and apartments it is also possible to attract, for example, more families, more shops or more elderly people. Apart from restructuring strategies, authorities can set out strategies to persuade people to move into the neighbourhood or to move out of it. Improving the infrastructure – services, business, access, streets and the green areas – is also a way to become more attractive. Sometimes authorities draft regulations to be able to carry out a restrictive policy in not accepting certain target groups in a neighbourhood.

2   Adequate and alert public and semi-public services. Most residents' complaints are generally about maintenance (rubbish, dog dirt, graffiti) in the community and the lack of input by all kinds of services (police, social workers, civil servants) in reaction to questions, comments and requests. Alert housing associations, schools and public services are creating trust and satisfaction. In deprived areas, services are sometimes poor as well. Adequate actions of professionals contribute to more trust and satisfaction.

3   Improving participation and interaction. A range of research indicates that participation of citizens in volunteering activities, in informal care and social networks, in democratic processes and in associations and institutions contributes highly to a more positive perspective on the community and contributes to a higher quality (perceived and actually) in different fields, such as safety, economic activities, health and wellbeing (Jacobs 1992, Putnam 2000). Improving participation is improving interaction. Interaction between people from different backgrounds is often a productive way of improving trust and mutual relationships between ethnic conflicting groups.

4   Improving the physical, economic and social infrastructure. Safety (actually and in feelings) and attractiveness of communities can be promoted by changing the physical infrastructure. It can be done easily by interventions such as improving street lighting, traffic lights and convenient and accessible recreational areas. Economic activities in the community can be promoted by enabling policies for business and an attractive social infrastructure through community schools, leisure activities, social services, child care and community centres.

The list of strategies is not complete and debatable. We are lacking convincing evidence as to which strategies are most promising and successful. The costs of the strategies differ dramatically. However, combining different strategies seems more effective than to rely on only one.

Community work

Short history

The history of community work starts in the nineteenth century with community centres and is joined later by youth work, community building and communities that care. In recent decades social management, planning strategies, integration of physical, economic and social pillars are changing community work, embedding it more deeply in neighbourhood programming.

Community centres

As seen above, community centres as the heart of the local community were in fact already implemented by American immigrants in the eighteenth century. As a deliberate strategy, community centres in disadvantaged neighbourhoods were set up to bring people together by enabling all kinds of activities organized by and organized for the neighbourhood. Toynbee Hall (1884) was the first community centre in this respect and from then community centres spread over Europe rather quickly. Those centres were fully in the hands of volunteers from the community, and often referred to as the 'settlement movement' (Barbuto 1999). The settlement movement had connections in universities and persuaded students to live and volunteer in slum areas alongside local people. The International Federation of Settlements still exists as a global network. The movement spread from the UK to the US and Russia, where centres were set up in the early twentieth century and later closed down by the Tsarist administration (Valkanova and Brehony 2006).

Youth work

Another origin of community work were youth clubs and centres, starting half way through the nineteenth century and evolving into professional youth centres. Those clubs mostly aimed at marginalized young people and tried to help them overcome their marginality by social education, group work and skills training. After the Second World War youth club work became popular in Europe. In Germany, youth clubs were promoted by the Americans to educate young people in social orientation and behaviour and to prevent new mass youth movements from following the wrong banners. Later, playgroups, playgrounds and child care were included as part of youth community work on the one hand, and on the other, outreach or detached youth work, for example, street corner work, and programmes like 'Communities that care' aiming at community strategies for early offenders and risk groups to prevent them from becoming criminals (CTC 2008).

Community building

This stands for community organization or community work in the meaning of strengthening communities by empowering residents, promoting their interests, fostering participation, capacity building, urban planning and community management. Community building or community organization was quite popular in the US during the 1920s and 1930s and started in Europe mostly after the Second World War in the process of rebuilding society and communities. Community work and community organization became more disputed at the end of the twentieth century. It was seen as rather ideological and vague in its methods, and debatable in effectiveness (Dominelli 2004, Smith 2006). In England education for community work/building was no longer seen as an academic subject (Dominelli 2004). Lately, however, community organization is back on the social agenda and embraced again in most European countries. In fact, a new market for public and social administrators and all kinds of project and programme managers is emerging. In the US community-building professionals were mostly employed in the field of urban planning and social housing projects, and there is also a growing market in some Western European countries.

Community care

A fourth source for modern community work is found in social care. Under Margaret Thatcher in 1980s Britain care in the community or community care was promoted as an answer to the institutionalization of the mentally ill and the frail elderly and attempted to involve communities in care and to create caring communities. Care for the elderly, disabled, marginalized and homeless became part of community work. The idea of community care fitted in with the so-called Declaration of Alma Ata's (1978) definition of health care:

> Health care based on practical, scientifically sound and socially acceptable methods and technology made universally accessible to individuals and families in the community through their full participation and at a cost that the community and the country can afford to maintain at every stage of their development in the spirit of self-determination.
>
> (WHO 1978)

Definition

Like most words and concepts in social work, we are lacking an internationally recognized definition for community work. Most definitions of community work mainly connect to community organization. One of the already quoted definitions is:

> Community work is that portion of activity focused on bringing about social change with a set of working principles, namely: that the process is collective, participative; is social justice and equality focused; and employs a methodology which is empowering and liberating to individual participants and the community.
>
> (Chanan 1997)

Here community work is close to a methodology focusing on the ideas of emancipation and liberation. Viewed internationally, community work is more than a methodology, encompassing objectives, perspectives, methods and different fields of activities. The English 'Gulbenkian Foundation' defined community work as:

helping local people to decide, plan and take action to meet their own needs, helping local services to be more effective and accessible and taking account of interrelation between different services, forecasting necessary adaptations to meet new social needs.

(Smith 2006)

This definition is close to Thomas's definition: *'to help people to take action, development of social responsibility, communal coherence'* (Thomas, 1983). The capacity-building definition of Skinner (1997) is in the same direction but includes structure building:

Development work that strengthens the ability of community organizations and groups to build their structures, systems, people and skills so that they are better able to define and achieve their objectives and engage in consultation and planning, manage community projects and take part in partnerships and community enterprises.

Those definitions are broader than the Chanan definition but were also challenged as not broad enough and neglecting certain areas of community work. Regan (2007) pledges a redefinition of community work and community development as simple as 'any form of activity that happens in a local area'. Quite a similar definition is from Hardcastle and Powers (2004): 'Community work is the sum of practice of different actors in the community.' The problem of those last definitions in our feeling is that they are too broad and do not translate into strategies and methods. Finally, Payne (2005) speaks about community work as social work 'as concerned with evolving a more effective social order' and

To improve the fit between people and their environment by alleviating life stressors, increasing people's personal and social resources to enable them to make use of more and better coping strategies and influencing environmental forces so that they respond to people's needs.

Here community work is defined from the social work perspective and related to ambitions and goals.

I suggest community work as 'the contribution from social professionals, together with and geared to the local citizens, in strengthening social cohesion, social capital and social competences of communities and their residents'. In this definition community work is a goal-oriented concept related to a certain territory and restricted to the contribution of social professionals but directly connected to the residents. The overall interventions in a community belong to community policy; community work is defining the contribution of social professionals. Important fields of activities are the four roots (community centres, youth work, community care and community building) and the grey areas between social work and education (schools), social work and urban management and urban planning, social work and safety and security (police) and social work and activation of the labour market.

Social work roles, tasks and methods in community work

The interconnected field of community-based social policy and community work is a complex domain with rather different concepts and objectives. In this section, we will deal with the most important fields, tasks and roles of social workers in community work domains.

To endorse and promote participation and activation

Community work is concerned with empowering residents to participate. Maybe supporting participation is the core task of social work. In community work stimulating participation is mainly a process of bringing people together and supporting existing participative networks. It is important to distinguish different levels of participation.

1   Informal participation. Informal participation is about everyday life where people take part in each other's life, in educating their children, in taking care of the elderly, in helping a friend or neighbour, in having a social life. This social fabric is an essential resource for individual life and for communities. It is closely related to social capital as social network and trust (Putnam 1992, 2000). A first challenge for social workers is how to support and – if needed – to strengthen this social fabric and the informal participation. In particular frail elderly people, people with serious learning disabilities and people with mental health issues often have difficulties in acting in informal participation. People are sometimes very isolated and excluded. In community work volunteers and sometimes professionals try to get people out of this isolation by visiting them and inviting them to take part in meeting activities or voluntary work. Outreaching social work has developed a range of methods to reach isolated people, people who avoid contact. Another method in strengthening informal participation is to support informal care. Informal carers are sometimes overburdened and need some respite and support. A third method focuses on organizing events, courses and meetings in the community to encourage people to participate and to interact with other residents.

2   Voluntary work and civil society. In general, in discussing participation, voluntary work and civil society spring to mind. Experts and politicians believe that an active civil society creates a more healthy and productive society. An active civil society saves costs because volunteers are organizing activities in sports, culture, care, education, the environment, etc. Social workers can find jobs in voluntary organizations as supervisors, coaches and facilitators. Sometimes, special support agencies for promoting volunteering work have been set up. Volunteers often support professional institutions, for example, in hospitals, in schools, in residential care homes. In that case it is necessary that professionals support and facilitate 'their' volunteers.

3   Participation in the labour market or education system. In the labour market discourse, participation implies bringing people back into labour or education. Activation is a method to get people back to work. Social workers are regularly involved in 'activation work'. Activation work is sometimes related to the 'distance to the labour market'. Most people succeed quickly and without professional support in finding a new job. Some need more time and some support, and some need full professional support to re-integrate into the labour market. And there are people who never will be able to participate fully in the labour market but maybe find jobs in sheltered work places or voluntary activities. Close to participation in the labour market is participation in education or school. In all countries, we deal with problems of school dropouts and children playing truant, and sometimes social workers are expected to bring them back into school. Activation as promoting integration in the labour market, or education, is often part of community work. On a community scale, we are able to monitor people, to reach them and to activate them.

4   Democratic participation tries to get residents involved in local (and national) politics. In the social domain, participation is often seen as the effort to give residents a say in decision-making processes in their community and to give them a hand in implementing and carrying out social programmes and projects. Community workers enable and facilitate residents and make them more competent to promote their own interests and to have a say in community development. Sometimes community workers represent their constituency in policy-making processes. One of the problems of this kind of participation in the community is that many residents do not want to get into conflicts with neighbours and to speak openly in those procedures (Keller 2003).

Social (community) workers act on different participation levels. They facilitate and support informal, volunteering, labour and democratic participation.

Social education and social cultural work

Social education refers to the tasks of social workers to endorse, support, challenge and train people in improving learning ((multi)cultural) and social competences. Social pedagogy believes and argues that leisure time creates great opportunities for informal learning. In the streets, in the clubs, in doing things at home in front of the computer or television, (young) people learn and develop competences which are needed in society. In marginal districts, this social cultural learning has been the basis for setting up community centres and youth centres. A popular strategy in social work is to set up training, clubs, events that contribute to informal learning and semi-formal learning, like preparing for school, activating for the labour market, preparing for old age or preparing for integration. A special methodology is 'social creative work' or 'community art work'. Drama, music, dance, handicraft, art education, organizing events, are 'media' through which residents develop new competences. Social educators, social workers, 'animators', are recognized social professions with a methodology based on a process of designing, carrying out and evaluating activities. Rural community centres are centres without professionals. Local volunteers manage the centre and organize activities. Community centres in marginal districts are mostly more professionally based. Those local professionals take care of managing the centre, supervising and conducting volunteers, and in providing services and carrying out activities such as courses, consultations, and training and community events. A special branch of community work is youth work. Youth work is often based at youth centres, sometimes fully on a voluntary basis, sometimes staffed by youth workers. Nowadays, outreach youth work is quite popular. Those workers try to connect to certain groups of youngsters in the community who are perceived as troublesome. The youth workers aim to change the behaviour of those young people, for example, by engaging them in sporting activities and by looking for jobs for those young people and to intervene, if needed, in their private, family and/or peer group life.

Another field of social cultural work focuses on connecting social education to the formal education institutes, as we can see in pre-school education, after-school education, playgroups and playground work and in community schools. These social workers are sometimes employed by schools, and sometimes by a community centre or day care centre. Core competences of social cultural workers are planning and carrying out activities, courses, events, binding (young) people to each other and to networks and institutions, and to create and strengthen networks in the area of education.

Community-building work

Community-building work focuses on strengthening communities and their residents, mainly by 'capacity building'. In capacity-building, professionals identify problems and resources in the community and develop, together with residents, solutions to the perceived problematic situations. That is the core business of community building. The community is seen as a system with characteristics of a learning and working community. 'Networks', 'social capital' and 'social infrastructure' are important concepts in this approach. Networks are (loose) groups of people, or organizations or a mix of organizations and people, related to each other by some common interest. The nuclear family, a school, a business are not seen as networks. The extended family, a number of schools working together or a number of co-operating firms are indeed networks. Social workers identify and empower networks in complex cases in youth care, disabled, elderly or mental health care to support the person involved. To meet the need for more safety in the neighbourhood police, schools, youth workers, sporting clubs and citizens create safety networks. Networks are an effective way of coping with complex problems in the community. Trust, horizontal social and democratic functioning of communities and the quantity and quality of relationships (networks) are decisive. Capacity building asks for a feeling for how networks function and how to interfere in networks, how to create trust and to empower a neighbourhood and community. Capacity builders are very good in identifying resources and to match needs and resources. Most community workers focus on empowering the local residents in promoting their interests and taking responsibility for their neighbourhood. They often connect local residents and their interests to systems, such as social security, public services, schools and the labour market. Professionals are links between community life and societal systems.

Social management

Social management is close to community building. The emphasis is more on the formal processes. A social manager represents the authorities and takes responsibility for the policy-making process. Social management, as a profession, is rapidly increasing in the social sector, particularly in regard to marginal neighbourhoods and districts. Such posts are open to professionals with different backgrounds, mostly from public administration and social work. A social manager co-ordinates interventions and actors in the community, develops and implements localized social policies and takes responsibility for the process of development, decision making and deployment of social interventions. Social managers are employed within public administration or in social work organizations or in community councils or platforms, or function as independent professionals on a temporary basis. He or she brings actors together, creates mutual agreements and plans common action. Mostly the managers lack real power and are dependent on convincing power and political support and acceptance by the most important actors in the community. Actors are from the public sector, civil society and business and from different sectors such as housing, social care, welfare, police, schools, and public administration. Sometimes the co-ordinating activities embrace social, economic and environmental policies; sometimes they are restricted to urban planning or social welfare or to certain programmes, 'areas' or projects. Social management is highly involved in local social policy processes. Local social policy making is to split into the content (what and how) on the one hand and the process on the other hand. Social managers are sometimes responsible for drafting social policy documents, neighbourhood programmes and projects, action plans and tendering papers. These more content-related tasks ask for a specific expertise in social knowledge (theories, practice) and in drafting plans. In general, action plans are seen as co-productive activities, involving different actors. The other side of local social policy making is about the process. From social managers it is expected that they have the capability to bring people together, to give all actors a say, to look for compromises and to smooth the whole process of development, decision making and implementation. The key competence for social managers is to identify and to analyse the problem properly, to mobilize resources effectively and to connect actors adequately. The social manager does not solve the problem alone but lets different actors do 'their' work.

Case and care management

Case and care management occurs if situations are very complex and people and their networks are not able to cope adequately with the problems. In that case, a social worker takes over the managing role and takes care of proper intervention and co-ordination between different professionals. Owing to the policy of de-institutionalization and localization we find nowadays more complex cases in the communities. Frail elderly people, those with serious learning disabilities, homeless people and people with mental health problems often need permanent support structures and social services. We distinguish between: intervening case management, supportive case management, youth care management and outreach case management. *Intervening case management* is a short term intervention where concerted action is needed. *Support management* is long term continuing support for a person who needs (semi)permanent intensive support and care. The tradition for case work in social work is based on intervening case management and case therapy. Long term case management has been the domain for nurses and in a number of countries for social pedagogues but nowadays is often integrated in social work practice. *Youth care case management* focuses on social education within the family and child protection by guardians and social pedagogues through intervention programmes, such as Families First or family coaching and family conferencing. *Outreach social case management* occurs if people are avoiding any help, intervention or support but definitely need it, or if people are causing trouble and action is needed. One characteristic for case managers is that their starting position is a person or multi-problem family and from there they manage the situation by co-ordinating and supportive activities. Mostly case workers are based in specialized social care, social work or youth institutions. Case managers are not 'therapists' but professionals taking responsibility for adequate help and support mostly carried out by different social professionals. Competences for case managers are a mix of rather pragmatic and managerial competences, competences to connect different actors, to match the personal situation and the services, to analyse the situations, to design interventions and support strategies.

Information and consultation

A last position and approach is informing and consulting people who are looking for services and support and to inform and consult policy makers and professionals about the community and its residents. Due to the complexity of modern societies, it is needed to help people to get access to social services by informing them, guiding them and consulting them to find the right place and person. The one-stop counter or one-stop service is a popular approach to concentrate all information in a certain field or zone, such as social care or social education or public services and to match need and supply of services properly. From the social professionals in those services adequate knowledge about the law, regulations, existing services, and resources in the community and matching qualities are expected.

Community work research and local knowledge

'Think globally, act locally' is the often quoted expression from René Dubos (1972), cited in Eblen and Eblen 1994. It means that we live in a global world affecting everyday life but that people act locally. It is in the local community that we most experience daily life. The local community is an excellent place to identify social resources and social problems, to monitor people in need of support and to intervene in upcoming local problems. A modern social professional is a local researcher by definition. She or he should have the capacity and quality of character to identify what is going on, which problems and needs there are, what resources exist and what kinds of interventions, methods, services are available. Local knowledge is knowledge about residents, the physical, economic and social infrastructure, about perceived problems, about resources to use for improving the individual and collective (community) context. For local knowledge we need different kinds of data and researches.

1   Statistical data about demography, feelings, and perceptions of residents. Big cities usually have their own statistics. Community workers should be able to understand and to manipulate this kind of data. Quite often statistical information is used for indicators in defining problematic districts. Cities often publish comparative lists of best and worse achieving districts or neighbourhoods.

2   Knowledge of physical (housing, traffic, streets, parks) and economic (shops, offices, bars) infrastructure and its functioning. Many perceived problems and annoyances in neighbourhoods are in regard to traffic, green issues, bars and restaurants and illegal economic activities.

3   Information about the services operating in the community. A social mapping of the community is needed to get an overview of and insight in what kinds of services, professionals and institutions function in the community. Even more interesting is to analyse what kinds of interventions take place, in particular regarding troublesome problems, people and groups in the community. It happens that a whole range of professionals and services are aiming at a similar group of youngsters or a multi-faceted problem.

4   Information about human resources in the community. Here we identify and analyse the social fabric in the community and civil society (informal networks and voluntary work). In disadvantaged neighbourhoods the social fabric is often weak and damaged and a well organized civil society hardly exists. However, closer research sometimes discovers that there are strong networks and informal civil society activities; however, these are not always on the 'right' side. For instance, gangs often create strong support and identity for their members but push them at the same time into criminality. Human resources in the community are not abstract, but are living and recognizable people. A community worker should know most of them by name and should be able to involve them if needed.

5   Contextual knowledge and contextual research aims at analysing concrete situations and problems in the community. This is, in my opinion, the most important item of research. What is happening? What can be done, and by whom? It is about perception, feelings, perspectives, facts, about human behaviour and human relationships. The context is maybe a family, a street, a gang, a playground, excluded elderly or disabled residents, recognized inconveniences, long term unemployed people, etc. Community workers have the competence to identify, to analyse those contexts and to design paths to improve the situation.

Therefore, a social professional in community work should have the research competence:

1   to understand, interpret and manipulate statistical data about the community;
2   to be able to undertake social mapping of services and interventions in the community;
3   to analyse the physical and economic infrastructure;
4   to analyse the social fabric and human resources in the community;
5   to research contexts in the community.

Discussion and assignments

Discussion

- The first thing to discuss is the importance of the community. What are your ideas about the local community as a cause and/or as a resource for answering social problems from individuals and groups?
- Discuss the different definitions of communities and argue for one of the options (geographic, community of interest or idealistic).
- Discuss promising strategies. What is in your eyes the most effective strategy to strengthen and to improve a community?
- We have presented four levels of participation. Which one is in your opinion is the most important in community work? Why?
- And we have presented six different roles (endorsement of participation, social education, community building, social management, case and care management, information and consultation) for social workers and community workers. Which one appeals most to you? Why? And which one does not, and why?
- Do you agree that community research is an important skill for community workers?

Assignment 1

- Write a short history of your life in the community, in particular how important the community was for you and about how it has affected your life.

Discrimate between when you were between 8 and 12 years old and when you were between 14 and 18 years old.
- Discuss in small groups the impact of the community on your lives and report a few keywords about it.

Assignment 2

- Present a community work concept or method by Powerpoint and draft a short (3–5-page) document You can do it in groups of one, two or three people.
- Some suggestions:
    - community centre
    - youth centre
    - outreach work
    - community care
    - communities that care
    - mediation (in neighbourhoods)
    - care support
    - community schools
    - community planning
    - one-stop counter
    - community art
    - youth and sports

6   Other fields of activity

Introduction

In this chapter we will look a little closer at other main fields of social work. We are not mapping those areas extensively, but just looking roughly at the main fields of activities, at recent developments and in particular at new concepts and approaches based on activation and participation. The three main domains are youth work and youth care, long term care, and social case work on exclusion and poverty (Bie and Ewijk 2008).

Youth work and youth care

Integrated sectors, bridging competencies and integrative identities

Fragmentation and specialization in social education and youth care is obvious in most European countries (Cambridge and Ernst 2006). We find different systems, mental health, juridical systems, youth care, local youth support services, disabled youth care, often with weak links between the systems. Within the different systems, again, we find all kinds of specific services, methods and treatments. At the same time, this whole system of interventions, treatments, support and preventive activities is hardly connected to the school education system and the communities. In most countries the services have great difficulties to meet increasing requests for support and intervention at the local level, in particular in the field of youth care and dealing with youth gangs. Localization and de-institutionalization effects a double aggravation. In institutions the most complex and troublesome children are left, because the policy is to intervene as much as possible at home, within the family and at school. This increasingly selective policy for accessing young people in residential institutions hardens the social climate in the institutions, on the one hand and aggravates local youth policy in the communities because more children with serious problems are treated and supported in their own environment, on the other. In addition to that, youth care institutions are dividing their organization into small units in the neighbourhood. In many countries policy makers are looking for more coherence between the systems, for case and care management, for co-operation within in the communities, for gateways (agencies) for assessment and placements to improve the link from contact to treatment and the link between different professionals and different services. Currently, a revival of integrated, generalist, even holistic, strategies in the social domain is going on, as discussed in Chapter 5. Social educators and other social professionals are increasingly connecting micro, meso and macro domains in life by intervening in families, peer groups, schools, in streets and in leisure time.

In modern welfare states, however, the emphasis is much more on formal education than on social education such as raising a child in a coherent and co-operative community. In different European countries the education of children under six has been placed under the Ministry of Education (Sweden, Spain), making it obvious that the first interest is in learning achievements. Day care for children is often perceived as contributing to the labour market strategy by enabling both parents or single parents to work (EC 2005b). Actually, only in some countries, kindergarten and child care are fully regarded as the domain for social pedagogy (Denmark) (Hansen and Jensen 2004). Nevertheless, 'learning to learn' is dominating the official European social and education agenda and is regarded as an important asset in boosting the knowledge economy (Council of Europe 2001). We should balance learning to learn and learning to live. To live and to live together is highly complicated in modern society (Chapter 2, pp. 42–3). One of the greatest concerns is the problem of determining your life path and lifestyle, and to feel motivated for directing yourself. It is a necessary requirement to build up educational and social capital and to acquire suitable behaviour in different contexts. People have to live with different identities and in different communities. People are expected to be flexible and mobile. They need bridging competences and the competence to create a life with many connections and relationships (weak ties), with trust and the courage to take risks. Bonding within the family or a closed community, an inflexible identity and too strong prejudices are hindering people's development and integration and are even regarded as threats to modern society (Putnam 2000). Learning to live and to live together, therefore, should be in the foreground of bringing up children and young people and not be restricted to the private domain of family life. Modern catchwords such as social competences, cultural competences and social capital reflect the postmodern feeling. Social competences are about how to deal with other people, how to understand them and to cope with their (re)actions towards you. Cultural competences refer to the capacity to express yourself verbally and non-verbally, to build bridges between your own cultural background and the background of other people and your education. Social capital concerns the quality, strength and impact of your networks, including the quality of trust (people and systems) (Putnam 1993, 2000).

Reasons to invest in young people

There are several reasons to invest in children and young people.

1   They are vulnerable and need protection, care and attention. A supportive living environment contributes to a stable and balanced development.

2　Society invests in young people for its own sake and future. To invest in social and learning education is to safeguard sustainability and progress. A society needs a national and local human resource strategy to strengthen its economic and social qualities. Adequate human resource management is not only concerned with learning competences. It includes social climate, social competences and social capital as well. That is common knowledge in the big industries, and should be more recognized in the public and private domains.

3　The concern for criminal behaviour, for deviant behaviour and a whole list of mental health-related concerns, from addiction to anorexia, require investments and cohesive youth policy strategies. The media and politicians are highly sensitive to incidents and violent behaviour. Feelings of being unsafe depend most on the existing visible criminality, often associated with (black) young males (Wacquant 1999, Boutellier 2002).

Ecologic pedagogy[1] and integrated, contextual related approaches

Ecologic pedagogy starts from the idea that we should focus on a strong, supportive and challenging social environment for children and young people. It embraces school, leisure time activities, the physical environment, urban planning, public place management, safety, youth care, child care and so on (Winter 2000). Intensive youth care programmes and care for seriously disabled children belongs to this ecological domain as well (Crockett and Crouter 1995). We should integrate intensive care and intensive interventions close to home and if possible in the community. Successful programmes in this respect are, for example, 'Communities that care' and 'Youth at risk'. Ecologic pedagogy is based on a number of basic principles (Bronfenbrenner 1979, 1986, Germain and Gitterman 1980, Tolan *et al.* 1995, Dubois and Krogsrud 1999, Winter 2000).

1　Upbringing asks for a strong living environment that supports and challenges children and young people. A balance between protection, supervision and exploration is needed. Local authorities should develop a view and policy to empower and to enable strong living environments for children and young people. All sectors are involved: schools, leisure time activities, youth care, the police, physical environment, public space management, housing, traffic and so on.

2　Upbringing asks for harmonizing, mutual understanding and co-operation between different actors, such as parents, teachers, youth workers, social workers, the police, general practitioners, all kinds of volunteers in sports, arts, churches, etc. In cases of troublesome complicated youth problems all actors are needed to tackle the situation. It cannot be done by one actor – one specific service or sector – only. Co-operation is essential.

3　Ecologic pedagogy has a strong belief in the power and capacity of people and their networks. The first thing to do is to look for positive energy and human resources. The perspective is not on the problematic side but on the promising aspects in an individual, his or her network and community. If actors, with a common understanding and a positive attitude, work together, the best chance for success is there.

4   Ecologic pedagogy is locally embedded, anti-institutional and co-operative. The influence of this kind of thinking, fed by the increasing number and increasing severity of many youth problems and the incapacity of the existing systems to meet properly the needs, affects more ecologic-based approaches, integrating services and sectors and empowering participation of all relevant actors. The increase of community schools, projects for safe and liveable neighbourhoods, combined local centres for parents and children offering integrated youth care and parental support, underline this development.

Mapping the domain

Social work as far as children and young people are concerned is mostly called social education or (social) pedagogy. For children and young people, their world is mostly dominated by family and school. Friends, peer groups, playing outside and inside the house grow more important with age. Social workers or social educators are mostly not appearing in their world but sometimes they are needed to overcome temporary difficulties. In welfare states, we find a fine woven system of several social services, based on differences in age (children, youth and young adults), on different problems, in different fields of activities – such as mental health, the judicial system, youth care, child care, care for children with learning difficulties, leisure time activities for young people and family support – and with different methodologies and different methods.

Family support

Family support is often understood as material support by child benefits and social assistance. For a long time, additional benefits for large families were found in many countries. To a certain extent, support moved from the material to the immaterial, towards providing services for child care, promoting regulations for parental leave and care leave and strategies to combine work and family responsibilities (part-time work, flexible working hours). Those new policies were partly based on labour market policy to get more people (women) into the labour market and partly for pedagogical reasons (Ewijk *et al.* 2002). A third strategy in supporting families is to offer services in kind: information, consultation, guidance and supervision to support parents in bringing up their children. The idea behind those supportive services is the fact that complex societies are challenging children and families much more, whereas standardized answers are lacking (Crockett and Crouter 1995). Modern parents are thought to be more uncertain and more ambitious at the same time. Another argument is about the greater variations in family life: more single parents, more divorces, more remarriages, more migrant families, and so on. Those families have sometimes more difficulties in raising their children and adapting to the 'standard' expectations. Finally, modern family support is aiming at increasing the participation of parents in child care, in schools, in leisure time activities and in community care. Family support in all its aspects needs a concerted policy, bringing the different elements together. Family support in this broad and participative concept is one of the essential elements in ecologic pedagogy.

Child care

In European countries, child care, in the meaning of day care centres for pre-school and after-school children, is a fast growing professional field of activities. In the Nordic countries child care is for long an accepted phenomenon. In Southern Europe caring for children was mainly kept within the (extended) family. Today, all over Europe child care is a recognized field in the social domain and children start at a younger age and stay longer in child care. Different opinions and practices are found about the character of child care (pre-education, holistic pedagogical, labour market perspective) and the organization (market, public, mixed system, financed by the state or the parents or mixed), and about the level of professionals in child care; from people with few qualifications to graduate professionals (Cameron and Moss 2007).

Leisure time and youth work

Patterns of leisure time vary highly. The time spent in the street, in front of the computer or the TV, in sport clubs, in art clubs (music, dancing, drama) differs highly and is dependent on age, ethnic background, gender, education, economic position and personal history. It is often discussed to what extent leisure time needs to be structured, professionalized and supervised. Leisure time pedagogy is an existing field in social sciences. The concern for leisure time is the risk of peer group pressure, all kinds of temptations and risks (abuse, drugs and accidents), the worry of 'what is my child doing in front of the computer'. This is an uncontrolled area for many parents and is sometimes a real nightmare. The question for social professionals and social services is when and how to intervene in this leisure time domain. In welfare states a professional infrastructure of social services for children and young people in disadvantaged areas is quite common. Community centres and youth centres have a great influence in most urban areas all over Europe. Outreach youth work has become more popular, and in this field, sporting activities to activate and to attract disadvantaged youth are often used. A joint arrangement between schools and professional leisure time activities is found in community schools and is spreading quickly. Schools are expanding their domain by starting formal education earlier (from four or five years of age) and by extending the time children are in school each day (from 8.00 to 18.00). The tendency seems to be, in particular in cities where community control is less influential or non-existent, to keep children in schools and in supervised leisure time the whole day long.

Youth care

Youth care provides care for children and young people in trouble. Youth care is often provided in connection with schools (school social work), to youth centres and to communities, for example, a youth information centre or an agency for young people and families. All European countries have specific institutions for residential care or intensive intervention programmes for youth care at home. Those institutions are not part of the (mental) health system but are more geared towards training, supervision and group work. The imprecise border with mental health is drawn differently from country to country. In mental health institutions, an individual disorder or personal characteristic is seen as the main cause of the troublesome behaviour and therapy is the core treatment. A third element in youth care is the judicial system, starting from child protection and reaching (youth) imprisonment. The number of young people in the juridical system is increasing dramatically in many welfare states. The number of young people in mental health care is increasing as well. Depressive feelings and behaviour and other psychiatric disorders are found more frequently in children and young people than 50 years ago. It is conspicuous that the increase in troublesome behaviour interventions is rising in nearly all welfare states (Loeber and Farington 1998). At the same time it is not easy to find the right figures across the different fields of youth care and related to the overall number of young people. A fourth specific area of youth care in most countries is the care of (learning) disabled children. Here we find special institutions and special schools, or special classes in schools, to meet the social education needs and capacities of those children. Having these different fields in most countries, it is a problem how to assess, refer and compare adequately. We are lacking evidence-based knowledge on what kind of method, service or institution is best for which case (Resnick and Burt 1996, Konijn and Yperen 2003). Sometimes it is felt to be a problem that many children and young people are in complex situations who do not fit into the existing categories of disorders or who have combined problems (for example, learning disabilities and criminal behaviour).

Long term care

Understanding care

Care in an international context is a troublesome concept. It does not even have an appropriate equivalent in several European languages (Ewijk *et al.* 2002). Care as a professional field is quite underdeveloped in most countries. Caring activities are partly understood as being done within the family and partly as part of health care, mainly carried out by nurses. Actually, care refers to child care and youth care as well. Long term care, however, excludes at least child care and youth care and refers to a recognizable field of care for people with disabilities, frail elderly people and people with (socio)psychological and psychiatric disorders. Long term care implies professional care aiming at functions like support, activation, care services, treatment, sometimes housing as well. The character of (long term) care is highly dependent on the way we look at its 'clients'. It makes a great difference if the user is seen as a consumer or as someone to protect, or someone who should be taken care of by his family members or as an independent citizen (Kröger 2001, Hansen and Jensen 2004). Many professionals, policy makers and politicians have great concerns about the future delivery of this care due to a lack of funding and care workers (Cameron and Moss 2007). And even more important, they believe it is essential that people with social, mental, learning or physical disabilities are seen and treated as independent people and able to care for themselves as much as possible. Modern politicians are stressing the need for self-care and informal care. The whole strategy is focused on empowering people, challenging them to take their lives in their own hands, to strengthen networks and to develop people's own capacities and competencies (Cameron and Moss 2007). The care worker is a supporter, someone who understands the needs, wants and situation of the user and is in dialogue with them. Historically seen, the treatment of long-term care has developed from

1   isolation, putting people into closed institutions without any treatment and isolating them from their families and community;
2   protection, by taking care of them in safe but often remote institutions;
3   normalization, aiming at participation in and acceptance by society;
4   diversity, starting from acceptance of being different and at the same time empowering for participation and integration in society;
5   (Co)citizenship based on the concept of active citizenship and accepting their specific position and contribution to the society or community (Hansen and Jensen 2004, Ewijk 2006).

Integrated care

Support: the core element of social services

In care services supporting people in being full citizens is the core task. 'Support' as strategy and method is a specific way of thinking and acting in care. The starting point is the idea that the 'clients' are aiming for autonomy and independence as much as possible and in that they are supported by professionals to facilitate this autonomy (Wilken and Hollander 2005). The professional and the user are both focused on strengthening three types of networks to support the care user: the network of the family, the network of the community and the network of care, health, transport, housing and welfare providers. In this approach the objectives of care services are beyond the delivery of care products. They are broader and more challenging. Of course, nursing and concrete care services are part of a supporting strategy but wellbeing, activation, and assisting independence as much as possible are defining the direction and actions.

Combining the different actors

To intervene in difficult situations or to support users with serious disabilities, a network of acting partners is demanded. In care services we need combined actions in two ways. First, care policies require the collaboration of clients, informal carers, volunteers, professional services and authorities. In caring, most of the work is done within the family, often supported by friends and volunteers. In the long run, long term care is only deliverable when we bring together the capacity of different actors in the most sustainable mix. This combination of resources implies a balanced support from men and women, from different age groups, from different socio-cultural groups and today this balance is lacking in different respects. It is obvious in the gender perspective (Knijn and Kremer 1997). According to statistics men are a little more active in care at home nowadays. But at the same time we are confronted with a process where care within the family is partly taken over by services in elderly care, home care and care for the disabled. In those services over 90 per cent of the workforce is female. As a result, care is becoming even more gendered, and the same is true in education and health. People in need of care, education, support or health live in a highly female world. To get a more balanced system of combined actions, we have to rethink and to adjust the roles and responsibilities of all those different actors and the interplay between them.

Community care and integrated local-based care services

There is a lot of evidence to argue that we need a recognized more consistent branch of care (social) services. Starting from the idea that care should be delivered at home and in the communities and not in institutionalized care, we should de-compartmentalize the separate fields of different care and social institutions. We need a more open, flexible domain in which services, informal carers, volunteers, public authorities, private businesses, men and women, different age groups again and again create networks and combine their actions. For that reason, care-welfare-housing community concepts are becoming popular. They imply that the whole range of care services should be organized on the community (village, district) level ranging from home care to 24-hour care in a special housing unit. Those services are provided for different target groups, such as frail elderly, people with disabilities, the chronically ill and people with mental health problems. The idea of integrated care zones is comparable with the idea of ecologic pedagogical zones.

Mapping the domain

It is interesting to see how different countries have different structures in the field of long term care. In Denmark a broad and coherent social care domain and a recognized professional, the social pedagogue, is dominant. Danish experts prefer to speak about pedagogy instead of care. This pedagogical perspective connects child care, elderly care, care for the disabled, youth care, community care and community development (Cameron and Moss 2007). In most countries the care domain is divided into different compartments, each with its own institutions and professionals. This fragmentation of services and professions, however, is under pressure from the well known processes of deregulation, privatization, de-institutionalization and decentralization. In most European countries the boundaries between sectors and professions are blurring. Nevertheless, the most acceptable mapping of long term care is along the lines of elderly care, care for the disabled and mental health care. They refer to recognizable fields of activities aiming at a specific target group. At the same time, for all three of them we find locally integrated services like home care, shelter and relief care and voluntary and informal care.

Elderly care

Elderly care is split between nursing homes, homes for the elderly, home care and informal care. Nursing homes are based on medical treatment combined with care. Nursing homes nowadays are dealing with very seriously ill (for example, dementia), or very frail elderly, needing continuing supervision and care. Homes for the elderly, residential homes, service centres and sheltered accommodation for elderly are supporting and caring elderly who are no longer able to live on their own and want to live in more sheltered surroundings. Home care supports elderly people who are able and willing to live in their homes with (some) professional support. In modern care policies home care has been promoted and expanded and if needed it is more intensified. It is assumed that it is more convenient for elderly people to live at home and presumably it is a less expensive service compared with a nursing home or service centre.

Care for the disabled

Care for the disabled covers a whole range of fully different disabilities. Many disabled do not like the label of being disabled or handicapped because of its negative connotation. A first essential division is between the physically and learning disabled. A second division is between disabilities in seeing, hearing, speaking versus other physical handicaps. A third difference is between disabilities from birth and disabilities by accidents and chronic illnesses. Fourth, we find all kinds of combinations and overlapping disabilities. Finally, a disability can be distinguished at different levels, for example, among learning disabled we are used to categorizing them in different 'classes', regarding the assessed intelligent quotient. Therefore, we find a large number of different services and institutes for people with a disability. All over Europe de-institutionalizing is going on in long term care and in the Nordic countries there is hardly any residential institute still in existence. Care is for many disabled people not the most important service. They require more accessible transport, more accessible schools and work places, more accessible public spaces and 'to be seen and treated as citizens'. Care is just there to support them on a level playing field with other citizens.

Mental health care

Mental health has a number of similarities with care for the disabled. There are numerous mental disorders and many people suffering a mental disorder are not diagnosed because they do not fit into the existing classifications of mental disorders. Most mental disorders as such are much less recognized and accepted in society compared to learning and physical disorders. In mental health de-institutionalizing is going on as well, and the current trend is to deal with mental health problems by intensive day programmes and by strengthening networks in the communities. To accept mental disorders and to learn to live with them is quite often a more promising approach than curing and continuing treatment of the disorder. For that reason, activating care is becoming a more accepted and respected area in mental health.

Social case work, exclusion and poverty

Poverty and exclusion: clarification of terms

Social work has a long tradition in fighting poverty and overcoming exclusion with continuing ambiguous feelings (Dubois and Krogsrud 1999, Payne 2005). In society we find two opposite positions in the debate on poverty. The first position is that supporting the excluded is just a drop in the ocean because the cause is not in the excluded person or group but in an unjust world (Humphries 2006, Price and Simpson 2007). On the other side of the spectrum, the poor are blamed, because they are not willing to participate and to behave themselves in a socially acceptable way (Hayes 2006). However, most problems have more complex backgrounds and poverty and exclusion are highly related to the context. We will look a little closer at the different explanations regarding exclusion and poverty. But first, we should clarify poverty and exclusion because they are not fully overlapping. Not all poor people are or feel excluded. Sometimes poverty is temporary and the poverty is not hindering the person to participate in society. Quite often poverty is attached to a certain period in life. Another thing to consider is the definition of poverty. Generally, poverty is defined in terms of a certain percentage of the average income in a country. Countries with a flat tax system have fewer poor people but in a poor country they are in fact real poor and in a rich country they are definitely poor but not that poor. A well known international criterion is the one and two US dollar income per day. Over 20 per cent of the world population has an income of less than one dollar a day and 40 per cent below two dollars (UN 2006, ICSW 2006). The figures have improved in the last ten years, mainly due to economic progress in China and India; on the other hand in Africa and the Black Sea area sometimes a dramatic impoverishment has occurred. In debating poverty, we should be aware if we are speaking about the very poor in the poor countries or about the relative poor in the welfare states. And to conclude, relative and absolute poverty definitions are still lacking a precise description of poverty. Poverty itself is a multidimensional concept (Mkandawire and Rodriguez 2000). Exclusion, on the other hand, is not by definition bound to poverty. Sometimes the not-poor can be excluded, for example, certain groups of immigrants, ethnic minorities and mental health patients. Exclusion is used in many different connotations, sometimes referring to socio-economic indicators in most cases, and sometimes associated with certain groups, such as immigrants, drug addicts and homeless people, and sometimes even in the meaning of being excluded from information technologies, is the new divide (Neil 2002). I suggest exclusion as 'non-participation in society and/or non-acceptance and recognition by the society'. Society stands for labour, education, civil society and its communities together.

Different explanations for poverty and exclusion

Roughly speaking, there are four groups of arguments explaining poverty and exclusion.

1   Exclusion and poverty as an outcome of a societal or political system. Nearly every societal system is based on a mechanism of inclusion and exclusion. Traditional societies have strong inner and outer perspectives, meaning that the group ties are strong and exclude other groups. In all cultures we find the powerful and the outcasts. Apparently, societies are apt to discriminate between different groups related to gender, ethnicity, tradition, age, disabilities, behaviour, etc. In the capitalist system competition is an important drive for economic growth. It implies winners and losers. Communist states did not succeed in establishing a real inclusive society either. Exclusion and poverty have always been there and societies are systems with exclusive mechanisms. This does not imply that every political system is equivalent to each other. Certain political systems are more promising in overcoming exclusion than others, but we are lacking convincing evidence to see which social-political system achieves best. The fact that injustice is inevitable is not suggesting that injustice should not be challenged. However, for explaining exclusion and poverty, it is true that political systems are an essential factor in creating exclusion and poverty.

2   Exclusion due to human excluding mechanisms and excluding actions. The first explanation focuses on societal and political mechanisms related to a state or states together. We are talking now about human behaviour and relationships and about culture. 'Mechanism' suggests that people are often not intending or aiming for discrimination and exclusion but the process of exclusion goes on outside the awareness of people's reflection. Within the framework of cultural history and existing patterns, people construct their own reality, their own beliefs and perspectives, partly unintended and unplanned. Inclusion and exclusion, connecting and disconnecting, are in human nature and in each culture.

3   So far, we have discussed exclusion and poverty as an outcome of societal structures and human interaction, partly as mechanism, partly as intentional. However, people are not only victims and exclusion is not always only an outcome of a mechanism of exclusion by others. It is fair to ask to what extent excluded and poor people could escape poverty or could participate in society by their own actions and under which conditions. Social professionals have an essential task in this respect. They are not the powerful change agents of

societies and cultures, but they can contribute to empowering people, to bridge, to ease access, to change to some extent institutions and social systems. People need to strengthen their social competences and social capital. Competences are partly internalized dispositions by personal biographies and biographies of families or groups (Bourdieu 1979) and partly qualities to learn and to develop. Social capital is the strength and quality of the networks people and communities dispose of. Competence and social capital is, to a certain extent, to develop and to strengthen, that is the optimistic basic principle of social work. In welfare societies many of the poor and excluded can be considered as victims of excluding mechanisms and actions in society and communities *and* by lack of educational, social and cultural competences and social capital and a basically positive attitude to active citizenship.

4   A fourth cause for exclusion can be found in mental disorders or dramatic events or disasters. Without doubt, many people have difficulties in coping with daily life and hide themselves away. Dramatic events and traumas can freeze or paralyse people or drive people away from relatives, housing, jobs and their community. Some people choose explicitly an excluded way of life. The approach of those excluded asks for a mix of empowerment strategies, networking, and more supportive and maybe therapeutic interventions and of course material support.

Mapping the domain

Case work and case management

The first domain is the case work of social workers in public services or NGOs, providing assistance to individuals or families in need. In many countries social workers represent the authorities directly. Their discretion has been defined by their public task to be fair and to help the needy. In this field, material and immaterial help go closely together, albeit often split over different professional groups. In complex situations a case worker changes into a case manager, taking over regular daily tasks and partly temporarily organizing someone's life. In other countries social services are more independent and are aiming less at inspection and more at activation strategies.

Rehabilitation

Another classic field is the rehabilitation of ex-prisoners or other temporarily fully excluded people. Social workers help them materially (housing, employment, education) and immaterially by empowerment, listening, providing information and strengthening networks.

Sheltering and supporting the homeless and other excluded

Sheltering services, counselling and supporting people who are homeless, addicted to drugs, battered, runaways and so-called borderliners is another social work domain. Partly it is getting people out of their situation. In other cases it is just helping them to cope with their situation. Sometimes people are under treatment by mental health services and social workers are there to provide more pragmatic help.

Multi-problem approach

A specific area of many social workers is involvement in supporting families entangled in a whole range of problems, like unemployment, abuse, divorce, serious conflicts with children, criminality, debts and/or serious health problems. In this context, a step-by-step approach is needed and a working together of different services and sectors (police, social assistance, youth care, etc.).

Integration of immigrants and asylum seekers

In most countries the political and media attention on problems with immigration is a recent phenomenon. The political climate has changed in recent years, because of growing tensions (9/11) and the number of people from abroad coming to European countries. For that reason many social workers felt themselves to be more and more in the role of carrying out strategies of supervising, expelling and providing inadequate social services (Hayes and Humphries 2006). On the other hand many social professionals are brought into action for reconciling different groups, to empower migrants to integrate into the host society and to fight against discrimination and exclusion.

Therapies

A particular area of social professionals is acting as a therapist, mostly (in the field of social work) as front line therapists for people with serious psychosocial problems. In countries like the US many social workers are similar to psychologists and identify themselves as (socio)therapists or clinical social workers. The emphasis is on regular therapeutic sessions. Art therapists try to get people into action by using drama, music, film, video, etc. Conflicts within families, between neighbours or in neighbourhoods are often solved by mediation. A recent new way of acting in problematic situations is to bring all the people involved together and to ask them to discuss solutions and to work together to get the problems solved, for example, family conferences.

Discussion and assignment

Discussion

* Do you agree with 'ecologic pedagogy'? What are arguments for and against it?

- What is your idea about the role and responsibility of the family in long term care?
- Do you think that most poor and excluded people in your country are victims of the system and excluding mechanisms or that it is more of a lack of competences or self-exclusion?

Assignment

Map the main structures in youth care, long term care and support for the poor and excluded in your country or city. Maybe you can create three groups to map the different areas. Compare your findings with the overview in this chapter and look for differences and similarities.

7 From assimilation to intercultural competences

A challenge for social work

Jürgen Nowak and Hans van Ewijk

Introduction

Over past decades, Europe has been intrigued and confused by its diversity. In all fields of social work, dealing with diversity is an issue, and often conceived as quite a problematic one. In this chapter we argue for interculturalism as a basic approach and attitude to diversity. Interculturalism tries to reconcile multiculturalism and integration to a concept of respecting diversity but rooted in a European tradition as well. The chapter starts with a short historic overview on migration and migrant theories. In its second section we will discuss intercultural social work.

Migration and migration theories[1]

Economic discourse

In general people migrate for better living conditions or for reuniting with their family or partner. Refugees have hardly any choice: they have to leave their country for their own safety. Migration is as old as humanity but its character has changed through the ages. The impact of globalization in our days is enormous. The mobility and the global economic ideology of free movement of capital, goods, industries and, to a certain extent, people has changed the perspective dramatically. In economic studies, attention was drawn first to low skilled migrants moving from poor countries to the welfare states. Migration was perceived from the perspective of the Western world and seen as a mainly economically driven continuing flow of poor people from South to North, from East to West. This process was driven by Western labour markets and created new opportunities for the poor in poor countries. In more recent studies the perspective has inverted. Welfare states were assumed to lose their interest in low skilled labour, exporting their industries to the East and South, and to gain interest in highly qualified people from poor countries. This thesis is debated at the same time and maybe the two things are happening simultaneously. The Western world still needs low skilled labour, in particular in social services (care), in cleaning and other service industries and therefore a certain flow of immigrants is inevitable. And, indeed, the Western interest is moving into the direction of engaging high skilled migrants. As Saskia Sassen made clear in her study *The global city* (1991) it is not only a movement from poor to rich countries. As a matter of fact, a dominant trend is the creation of big cities where, on the one hand, capital and knowledge concentrate and the poor are engaged in service industries and, on the other hand, the cities 'rob' the county of its natural resources, creating an impoverished world outside them. In this respect, there is hardly any choice for the poor between being impoverished in their original residence or impoverished on the outskirts of the big cities. Along with this economic discourse is the idea of a dual labour market. A dual labour market creates a nearly unbridgeable split between the market for qualified people and the market for unqualified people and some other groups, such as the long term unemployed, people with serious disabilities or mental health problems (Han 2007).

Socio-cultural discourse

Migration is perceived as a societal and scientific problem from the 1920s onwards, starting in Chicago (Han 2007). Until about 1880 US immigrants were dominated by people from Western and North Europe, most of them being Protestant and motivated to start a new life in an 'empty' country. From the 1880s onwards, a new influx of immigrants came from Southern Europe and were perceived as threatening by the first immigrants, even leading to a selective and restrictive immigrant policy, favouring the Western and Northern immigrants. It raised questions about the problematic side of migration in the US. Until the twentieth century immigration was a common enterprise to build up a new country. It was perceived as the creation of a new nation. The well known 'melting pot' theory originated from the idea that people from different countries and cultures create a new world in a new country (Han 2007). The first migrant studies and theories developed the assimilation concept. This theory explains immigration as an individual effort to integrate into a new country, based on collective aims and ideals. In this process of assimilation different phases are recognizable: starting with communication and contact making and from there to a stage of competition and conflict, and then, finally, accommodation will take place. Accommodation is the acceptance of the new situation and the will to integrate into the new society. People have found firm ground and from there assimilation is the last stage, referring to a full implicit integration process (Han 2007). The first basic theories were later worked out, and deepened by Milton Gordon (1964). He recognized the different ethnicities, the role of religion and the economic political structures as important elements in the integration into the new country rather than assimilation theories. He put three ideological concepts at the heart of the assimilation process: Anglo-conformity, melting pot and cultural pluralism. An interesting position was taken by Shmuel Eisenstadt who focused on Israeli immigrants being nearly all Jews, sharing their ethnicity, but from many different countries, from Portugal to Russia, from Ethiopia to America. Eisenstadt used 'absorption' as a key concept. Absorption assumes a two-sided process between the immigrants and the host country. In absorption, the strategy, the willingness, the attitude of the host population is as essential as newcomers' actions and reactions (Eisenstadt 1954).

In the 1960s ethnic coloured groups in the US protested openly and vehemently against assimilation because they were disappointed in the outcomes of the 'melting pot' concept. They felt, and actually were, discriminated against and they believed in their own power and ethnic identity. Against assimilation they fought for recognition of being different as a fact and as a choice. Here started the multicultural concept. The strength of a society depends on its capacity to give room to diversity and to connect different ethnicities at the same time. It was the end of the big melting pot ideal as the creation of a new shared American identity, replacing it with the ideal of a great diversity of American identities. The multicultural discourse developed into a whole array of studies of different ethnic groups, re-evaluation of indigenous ethnic groups and paying attention to different positions coloured by gender, age and class, even expressed in the new word 'ethclass' (Han 2007).

Transnational regionalization

Immigrants have been seen as temporary workers or permanent settlers. Recently, much more attention has been drawn to migrants who are combining living in the home country and in the new country. They live their lives in two different countries, being different in both countries at the same time. It is the creation of a transnational ethnicity not as a temporary situation but as a permanent and desired situation. In economic terms, modern mobility enables those multi-local and trans-cultural connections and commitments. However, regionalization has an even greater impact on this 'de-territorized' way of living. The creation of regions such as the EU, ASEAN (South East Asia), NAFTA (North America) enables a nearly full free movement of people between the member states within the region. Those de-localized communities used to be found under the very rich, living as expats in the big cities, or as pensioners on the warm coasts of Southern European countries, but are now to be found everywhere. Migrants are, thanks to physical and virtual mobility, able to keep permanently in touch with the country of origin and vice versa. Like multinationals, those multinational-migrant-communities are changing the nation state. What about the passport or national identity? Should people living partly in one and partly in another country make a decisive choice between them, and why? What about democracy, voting and being voted? It is challenging the concept of national identity and citizenship, and new transnational and intercultural mechanisms and competences are developing. In Khagram and Levitt's words:

> By transnational, we propose an optic or gaze that begins with a world without borders, empirically examines the boundaries and borders that emerge at particular historical moments, and explores their relationship to unbounded arenas and processes. . . . A transnational perspective is also, therefore, a way of understanding the world, a shared set of questions and puzzles and a different expectation.
>
> (2008: 5)

Diversity in Europe

'Unitas multiplex', or '*Unity and diversity*', in Europe is an official slogan of the European Union (Morin 1988). It implies that many different nations with a great and broad diversity in cultures, languages and regional particularities are an accepted reality in the European Union. All those countries share a tradition, interpreted and defined by the unique historical heritage. This heritage started with antiquity, Greek philosophy and arts, and the Roman law and the building of an empire. A second legacy is in Christianity, with its different denominations, Catholic, Protestant, Orthodox. The third one is on influences of humanism, the Renaissance and the Enlightenment, characterized by their belief in progress, in respect for human beings and the 'thinking' power of people, reasoning. It depends on the personal point of view if people are emphasizing the differences or the commonalities of all European countries but in both cases this diverse and common Europe can be analysed and conceived as a 'network of interdependencies' of economic, social, linguistic and political relations within Europe in the last two millennia (Nowak 2001). However, this picture or idea has rapidly changed in the last four decades. The socio-economic differences within Europe, the creation of a common market and the increasing mobility from outside and within the EU have caused multiple processes of migration in and from European countries. In 2006 alone, over 3 million migrants were moving from one country to another, 60 per cent of them from outside the European Union (Eurostat 2008). In the long run, the number of migrants within the EU is increasing and from outside stabilizing or decreasing. Most migrants came to Spain, the UK and Germany in 2006. Relative to its own population Luxembourg was getting most newcomers. From outside the European Union most immigrants came from Morocco, Ukraine, China and India (Eurostat 2008). Not only does Europe as a whole have a great diversity but nearly all European countries have to cope with an increasing diversity of different cultures, languages and mentalities among their own residents. Most of the national European states are now multicultural societies, referring to the fact that many new residents have their roots and backgrounds not in the European heritage but in Arab and Muslim traditions, in Hinduism, Buddhism and all kinds of African and Asian cultures.

Two cases and a European (statistical) overview

Statistical figures and case studies are showing a clear picture of this new diverse reality in Europe. We provide just two examples and some statistics to give an impression of the migration impact on Europe.

Germany

Germany became a multiethnic society after the Second World War. The first so-called guest workers were invited in 1955 from Italy and later on from all the Mediterranean countries to fill the need for cheap labour by the West German economy. The term 'Gastarbeiter' (guest worker) was coined in order to avoid the old term 'Fremdarbeiter' (foreign workers) which was used during the Nazi era for 7.8 million enslaved persons deported to the Third Reich to maintain the agricultural and industrial weapon production. After the Second World War the percentage of foreigners was constantly increasing from 1.2 per cent in 1961 to over 4.3 per cent in 1970, 7.0 per cent in 1990 to 8.9 per cent in 2007. Nowadays the official number of foreign passport holders is 6.75 million (2007). Ahead in the ranking are the 1.7 million Turks, then 528,000 Italians, 385,000 Poles, 331,000 Serbs, 295,000 Greeks and smaller numbers of Croats, Russians, Austrians, Bosnian, Dutch, etc. (Federal Statistical Office Germany 2009). As far as the official numbers are concerned, it is often the case that much depends on definitions and the data collection. This statistical picture changed dramatically three years ago, astonishing nearly everyone, especially the political elite and the mass media. What happened was that the results from a different research project from the same office were published. The Federal German Statistical Office published the data of the micro census of the year 2005. It was the first time people were asked in interviews about the migration background of the last two generations of their family. The result was that out of 82 million inhabitants 15.3 million have a so-called migration background, that is approximately 18 per cent of the population with a non-German background, much more than was assumed before. In the last 50 years in Germany the names coined for this non-German population were changing regularly, starting with 'guest workers' (1960–1980), changing to foreign citizens (1980s) and later into migrants or immigrants (1990s) and currently ending in 'citizens with a migration background'. It shows the awareness and difficulties in avoiding discriminatory labelling.

Spain

In its history of the last five centuries Spain always has been a country of emigration. After the conquest of South and Central America (1492) there was a huge migration to Latin America and then after the Second World War to the more industrialized countries of Europe, for example, to France and Germany. In the last decade the opposite has happened: Spain has become a country of immigration from Eastern European countries and additionally reimmigration from the Latin American countries, and 'sun-seeking' elderly people from Britain, the Netherlands, Germany and other Western and Northern European countries. The distribution of the migrant population in Spain by nationality nowadays is as follows (Monivas and Ciot 2008: 59).

Overall	4,482,568
Moroccans	576,344
Romanians	524,995
Ecuadorians	421,384
British	314,098
Colombians	258,726
Bolivians	198,770

The total number is more than 20 per cent of the Spanish population. A new diversity from outside is added to the internal cultural diversity of Castilian, Catalan, Galician and Basque people.

European countries in an overview

Spain and Germany are just two cases but are highly recognizable for the EU member states in the West and South. Each country has it own characteristics, like France with high numbers of North African migrants, often from former colonies and a fierce debate on assimilation or multiculturalism, and the UK with a long history in immigration from Asia and former African colonies. In Eastern European countries diversity is increasing but emigration is perceived more as a problem and fewer people from outside Europe are emigrating to those countries. However, many people from the former Soviet republics (Georgia and Belarus) are moving to East European countries. The diversity problem is quite often affected by the past, such as Russians living in the new independent former Soviet states or mixed populations in the former Yugoslav states. The Nordic states have lower figures of migrants from outside Europe.

Table 7.1 European OECD countries and their percentage of migrants (OECD 2009).

Country	%
Germany	8.9%
Luxembourg	36.9%
Switzerland	20.5%
Austria	8.5%
Belgium	8.2%
Greece	7.0%
Ireland	5.9%
France	5.6%
Sweden	5.3%
Denmark	5.5%
United Kingdom	4.5%
Norway	4.3%
The Netherlands	4.2%
Spain	3.8%
Finland	1.7%

Former colonial powers like France, the United Kingdom and the Netherlands have low figures in this OECD overview, because many of their immigrants from former colonies have the citizenship of their country of residence.

The enlargement of the European Union to the East in the years 2004 and 2007 has its particular impact on internal European migration. Between Western and Eastern Europe there still exists a gap between living standards, causing a migration process from the East to the West with consequences for both sides. The EU strong economic and social position makes it attractive for people from all over the world looking for improvement of their situation to move in this direction. On the other hand, the EU is considering more and more restrictive policies to prevent an increasing influx of immigrants, leading to the fortress Europe approach, referring to a Europe with internal open borders but an external, more restrictive border.

Intercultural social work

The discourse

In the last decade a new term 'interculturalism' has emerged as a controversial topic in the discourse of social scientists and social workers. The concept behind the word is answering the discourse from assimilation to multiculturalism, and from the immigration perspective to the transnational and transcultural perspective. The recognition of diversity or pluralism in the multicultural discourse took place within the debate about Western progressive thinking, starting in Greek and Roman times, through Christianity to the Enlightment and forward to a scientific and rational world creating the best life for everybody (the Modern World) changing into a global thinking of contextualization, constructivism, cultural relativism and a fundamental doubt about a progress ideology (the Postmodern World). The risk of postmodernity and multiculturalism is the creation of absolute relativism and underestimating the deep-rooted basic economic structures of post-modern society, determining social life to a great extent: 'L'hypothèse multicultur-aliste absolue est aussi absurde que celle de l'homogénéité culturelle d'une ville ou d'un pays. Les relations interculturelles sont la seule réalité'[2] (Touraine 2005: 247). Interculturalism is based on the recognition of differences *and* similarities between cultures, groups and individuals. Interculturalism tries to overcome absolute relativism by emphasizing that society needs connections and a certain consensus, respecting dissensus at the same time. Interculturalism is the recognition of differences and similarities in a changing contextual historic framework. It is open to differences and change as for what is shared within the historic context of the country and region. Cultures and people are rooted in a territory but those territories are open territories and transformable; that means giving the new influx room for becoming co-citizens in the history to come. Such a mutual respectful position is the beginning of an empowerment strategy. Migrants or minorities should not be considered as 'deficit' persons who always need our care and support. They have their own resources which have to 'be awakened' and to be transferred into the society.

Intercultural competence

Interculturalism as a basic approach to ethnic diversity has been operationalized in intercultural social work and intercultural competences. In Germany, all universities have to include the dimension of 'intercultural competence' in social work education. Gradually, a certain shared concept on intercultural competences in this discourse has arisen. Overlooking the resources, we identified the following elements for intercultural competences (Gaitanides 2003, Handschuck and Kalwe 2004, Freise 2005):

- Openness: to new understanding, new insights, new backgrounds, new demands.
- Communication ability: to listen to each other carefully and respectfully recognizing the different backgrounds and contexts.
- Empathy: willingness and ability to empathize with the attitude of another person and to understand him or her.
- Multi-perspective(ness): consideration of a problem from different angles, including analysing majority perspectives, and minority perspectives, including differences in ethnicity, gender, age, lifestyle, etc.
- Self-reflection: a critical and constructive exchange of thinking; evaluating and preparing social action in the perspective of difference and affinity.
- Tolerance of ambiguity: to have the courage to cope with insecurity and unpredictability.
- Flexibility: to adapt to new contexts and new users without prescriptive models and with room for discretion.
- Conflict capability: to speak freely without threat of violence and unnecessary power and to intervene properly in situations full of tension, aggression, fear and discrimation.
- Knowledge about the background (history, religion, lifestyle, values) of different ethnic groups and differences within those groups.
- Knowledge about the social construction of race, ethnicity and nations.
- Knowledge of the social meaning and function of stereotypes and prejudices.

The importance of knowledge

The risk in competence approaches is to be too implicit about knowledge. To communicate properly with the right sensitivity is not good enough in intercultural social work. In understanding the other, substantial knowledge about the person against her or his economic, psychological and cultural background is necessary. Culture is something people appropriate by learning and experiencing. The learning elements are always present in culture. Stories are told from generation to generation. Religions ask for learning and numerous other aspects and elements. Therefore, culture is (at least partly) learnable and should be learnt (Pitkänen 2007). In social work, exploring the users' background within their context is an essential condition. Intercultural social work is even more complex because in many cases we lack personal experience in the cultural background of the other. The distance in language, culture, religion is usually bigger than encounters with users from the same culture and language. Intercultural social work asks for learning the substance of cultures and the differences between cultures and the cultural backgrounds of citizens. The cultural component in the background embraces elements like history and the personal narrative (life history), a feeling of, and practical knowledge for, religion, ethics and values, the role of family, community and social capital, the language (experiencing the gap between languages and difficulties in expressing oneself properly), the political background and maybe sensitive issues, and different aspects in attitude and common rituals in daily contacts. An intercultural social worker recognizes the discourse from assimilation to transnationalism and the critical political debates about migrants and is informed on theories and practice in social categorizing constructions of race, ethnicity, nations and cultures, on stereotyping, prejudices and discrimination. This implies a full programme of intercultural knowledge in social work education and studies. It is essential that in defining intercultural competence, the knowledge part in it is explicitly included. Intercultural competence for us is: to understand the other against her or his economic, psychological and cultural background within its own context and to connect to the other in a proper way, recognizing and respecting differences and similarities with an explicit knowledge about the substance of cultures and ethnic diversity. We use the word 'other' because the intercultural competence not only concerns the relationship between professional and client, but also relationships in the workplace. Intercultural social work concerns working in organizations as well.

Challenging social work

Interculturality is a multiple challenge for social work. We need a social work theory and practice which includes the intercultural, international and transnational perspective. Some more decisive and quicker steps need to be made. First, in the body of knowledge of social work, intercultural social work should claim its proper position in the front, and not be relegated to the corner of peculiarities and free courses. Social work needs a much more elaborated discourse on intercultural theories and practice. Second, intercultural social work should be implemented in adequate undergraduate and graduate courses. And universities and schools need much more exchange in developing those programmes in a process of shared learning. Third, social work practitioners should be supported, encouraged and challenged to enrich their experiences with deepening and broadening knowledge and to enrich the body of knowledge by exchanges and intervention to make implicit knowledge into a more explicit knowledge. Fourth, social work services should be more open to an intercultural organizational culture, for engaging social workers from different cultural backgrounds and supporting learning pathways for their workers in (intercultural) social work. Fifth, social work services and social work professionals should make an effort to be more accessible and recognizable from the different ethnic groups in societies.

Discussion and assignment

Discussion

In the first section of this chapter we presented different approaches to migrant studies in the economic and the social perspective. Do you agree with the emphasis on the transnational and intercultural approaches? Give arguments in favour or against.

At the end of this chapter the authors recommend that intercultural social work should be much more in the forefront of social work education and social work practice. What are your thoughts and why?

Assignment

Draft a small report on migrants and migrant strategies in your own country. What are the facts and figures (numbers) and definitions of migrants and which strategies regarding migrants are implemented and maybe discussed? Conclude with your opinion about the intergration politics in your country.

8 Social work as a profession, research and science

In this concluding chapter we will deal with some questions about professionalizing social work and on social work as a science. In the first section, we discuss standards, recognition of the profession, room for discretion, ethics, status and levels of functioning. The second section is on social work research, its characteristics and recognition, the different research fields and research competences.

Professionalization

Professionalization stands for the permanent effort to improve professional practice. A professional is a reflective practitioner who is able to use and apply scientific and practical knowledge in different contexts. This professional is in a continuous learning process, implicitly and explicitly.

Standards

To be accepted as a professional certain standards or expectations have to have been fulfilled:

1 A profession is recognizable, recognized and accepted as a professional field in society.
2 A profession is based on a recognized specific body of knowledge.
3 A profession is reflective by nature and his ample room for discretion.
4 A profession has a professional code or code of ethics.
5 A profession has a register.
6 A profession has a legal status (Banks 2006).

Some professions meet all those criteria, like doctors or lawyers. It is however debatable whether professions have to meet all these criteria. In postmodern societies flexibility in professional domains is expected and professions which are too rigid and not open to adaptation to political or managerial objectives are often discussed. It has become more usual to speak about professional domains or professional expertise and not to defend the profession as one which is too strong

(Banks 2006). In my opinion the first four criteria are most relevant, referring more to content than to formal procedures.

Recognizable, recognized and accepted

The problem with social professions is that in many countries and internationally a strong and clear overarching social professional identity is lacking. Most professionals in social work relate to their concrete function or specific profession, such as youth worker, art therapist, community worker, social pedagogue or social worker. As quoted before, social works seems to be 'a network of occupations' (Payne 2005). For the public, and for professionals from other domains (health, education and public administration) social work is quite often not regarded or perceived as a cohesive, professional field by lack of a clear profile and by lack of a recognized professionalism. The idea that social workers are substitutes for informal care and volunteers, 'just' taking care of certain family-related tasks is often found, particularly in countries in transition and countries with a less developed social work field (Ewijk 2007). On the other hand, internationally, a strong movement is going on to unify the different specific professions and educational fields under a shared umbrella and to profile social work under the ENSACT umbrella (2009). Thanks to the Bologna Declaration schools and universities for social professions are developing a more common 'language'. Social work as an international 'brand' is one of the outcomes of this process. In many countries social work has been recognized as a real profession with complex tasks and an individual professional autonomy (discretion) and the number of graduates with Masters degrees in social work is increasing rapidly all over Europe. In discussing privatization we noticed the eagerness of the European Union to privatize social services, being the second largest industry in Europe and one of the fastest growing ones. Social services in the broad sense are a highly interesting field for policy makers, economists and the public. They create a new area of feeling good, of improving neighbourhoods, of supporting the needy, of comfortable arrangements for people who can afford them and of solving social conflicts.

A specific body of knowledge

In fact, social work has an extended body of knowledge. Thousands of methods, an endless number of different practices, theories, functions, tasks and concepts are found. There are two major problems. The first one is that the body of knowledge is not very well organized and not overarched by a firm shared concept or theory or even a recognized framework. The positive thing is that the body of knowledge is fully developing and has a strong innovative and highly flexible character (Turner 2000, Scherer 2002, Thole 2002a). The second one is that the social work body of knowledge is much disputed and not often recognized by neighbouring fields (health, education, law) and in academic circles (social sciences). In this respect the social work body of knowledge is rather new and needs more depth, profiling and voicing.

Reflection and room for discretion

For me, the most characteristic aspects in professionalism is the professional quality to research contexts, to design strategies and concrete approaches, to answer the needs, the requests and the problems of citizens, to carry out the tasks properly, and to account for the results and outcome. A profession is in that respect by definition not fully standardized. A professional has to apply his or her body of knowledge in new situations again and again. One of the features of professionals is their room for discretion. Social professionals are by nature professionals in-between a whole range of dilemmas (Dominelli 2004, Payne 2005, Banks 2006). I present some social work dilemmas to illustrate this dilemma-oriented reflective practice.

1   The dilemma of conflicting interests, conflicting persons and conflicting actors. Social work is by definition trying to reconcile and to find a way out of tense situations. A social professional has to bridge gaps and conflicts between different interests, different opinions, different perspectives and different positions. The simple quote 'social professionals meet the demand of the consumers' is much too easy, because of this interrelational character of social work.

2   The dilemma of conflicts between systems and people. The social professional represents the public interest and is supposed to support the user at the same time. Real tensions are there if the public interest and the political objectives are felt as conflicting with the interest of the person or people involved. It is however too easy to state that social workers are always working for their users' interest.

3   To intervene or not. A social professional often feels the need to intervene but realizes at the same time the risks of an intervention. Family or authorities can press to act directly but the involved person is not willing and open to intervention. Suddenly, the professional dilemma can change into a professional failure because, before intervening, dramatic events take place: the killing of a child, a serious row between competing youth groups, maltreatment of a partner. Media and politicians are openly criticizing social professionals for ignoring or underestimating the problems or for intervening too late on the one hand, and at the same time blaming social workers for too much interference in private and civil society issues.

4   Conflicts between user values and personal values. People supported by professionals sometimes have ideas and feelings fully against the personal opinions of the professional, for example, regarding women, regarding migrants, regarding homosexuality, regarding what best can be done in a certain situation. It can be difficult to support people with great differences in values and norms. In modern days where answering the needs and requests of citizens is predominantly dominating the discourse, this tension between the social professional's own values and those of the client or consumer are felt even more strongly.

5   Involvement versus distance. Social professionals should be involved in their relationships with the users. The whole profession is about relationships and to win the users' trust. To support people, the social professional has to listen carefully, to open him or herself to the feelings, ideas and emotions of the other. However, distance is needed as well. First, it is necessary to make room for reflection and to analyse and transcend the perceived problems. Second, the social professional represents the public interest or common good and is not expected to be too one-sidedly committed to the client.

6   Confidentiality versus public interest. Social professionals hear and see a lot and sometimes they find information that can endanger other people in the family, in the community or even the whole society (terrorism, criminal activities, violence). Social professionals are expected to report about users deceiving authorities, about threatening conflicts or planned criminal activities. However, one of the professional codes is confidentiality and respecting privacy.

It is obvious that reflection and discretion are highly important for social professionals. They should be able to respond to users' needs, to public interests, to the law, to the objectives of the local authorities and their managers and to find their way in the best interests of users through the different dilemmas.

Professional code of ethics

In most European countries professional national codes of ethics for social professionals exist. Quite often we find different codes for different specific professionals in social work. Social workers as a professional group are maybe most advanced and precise in formulating their codes. On the international level social workers have an agreed code of ethics (IFSW 2009b). A difficulty in drafting a code of ethics is the concreteness of the ethics: how detailed should they be described? In the previous section we stressed the fact that professionals need room for individual autonomy and to adapt to the situation and to find their way through the different dilemmas. Too detailed and prescribed ethics are hindering professional discretion. As a matter of fact, a social professional should be able to reflect from metaethics. Metaethics is thinking about and reflecting on the application and meaning of ethics (Banks 2006). It is not just to observe ethics automatically. It is always applying them in continuously different, partly unpredictable, contexts. Therefore, in discussing codes of ethics we should deal with them in reference to the metaethical dimension.

Experts expect several positive effects of code of ethics (Dubois and Krogsrud 1999, Banks 2006). Ethical codes:

- provide practitioners with guidance in their daily work;
- make social workers trustful to the public;
- protect users from malpractice and abuse;
- make social professionals trustful to authorities;

- foster a common framework of understanding and professional behaviour;
- regulate and discipline the profession;
- protect professionals from litigation.

Some important ethics for social professionals are: respecting the right to self-determination, promoting the right to participation, respecting each person as such, identifying and developing strengths, challenging negative discrimination, recognizing diversity, distributing resources equitably, challenging unjust policies and working in solidarity (IFSW 2009b). Additionally, some more specific ethical codes for social workers are:

- to develop and maintain the required skills and competences to do their job;
- not to use their skills for inhuman purposes;
- to act with integrity;
- to work with compassion, empathy and care;
- to maintain confidentiality;
- to be accountable.

As you can see, those ethics are not precise prescriptions but always ask for interpretation and explanation of specific situations.

Register and legal status

In many countries social professionals are registered nationally, sometimes within the framework of a legal status by law. Sometimes registration is obligatory. In those countries, unregistered professionals are not allowed to practise as social workers, or at least participate in certain areas of social work, such as social work within a public service. Mostly, registration is voluntary and related to membership of a national association of social professionals. In both cases, requirements for registration are proof of adequate education, adequate professional experience and credit points for training. In Europe 165,000 social workers are registered in 35 different countries (IFSW 2009c). One of the debates is how to define social workers. You can find different registrations for social workers and social pedagogues.

Different levels in the workforce positions

The overall social workforce is divided into different levels. It is helpful to speak about professionals regarding those who hold a Bachelors degree or higher level qualification and about workers for the first three levels. Overseeing the level of workers and professionals together five different positions can be distinguished:

1   Assistants. Assistants in social welfare have little or sometimes no education in professional skills and competences. In particular, in home care we find many unskilled workers. In child care they can also be found, mainly assisting

better educated workers. They are assumed to work under direct supervision of better qualified workers.

2   Skilled workers. The characteristic of skilled workers (craftsmanship) is that they are well trained and skilled in a defined area of social welfare and a specific way of working. Many of them are found in social care, child care and among social pedagogues. They are assumed to work independently in not too complex contexts.

3   Professional generalists. Professionals are reflective practitioners and are able to deal with complex contexts and complex assignments. Their work is mainly in unstandardized settings and they have to find answers for new situations, needs and problems. Social professionals are predominantly generalists and front line workers found in all fields of activities. Social workers and most social pedagogues and community workers are operating on this professional level.

4   Specialists. Specialists are a combination of professionalism and craftsmanship. They are concentrated in a specific field (for example, youth care) or a specific task (for example, assessment) or a specific method (for example, video home training). Specialists are mainly found in offices (institutions, specialized organizations). Usually they hold Masters degrees and sometimes doctorates.

5   Scientists. Scientists in social professions are usually researchers or R&D staff members. They are rather rare in social services. In general, research institutes and universities employ them. Scientists and researchers hold Masters degrees or doctorates.

Different levels of functioning

Levels of position are based on levels of education and position in the social service. A different way of looking at different levels is in distinguishing levels of functioning in the professional career. Benner (1984: 13–34) created for nurses a well known scheme from novice to expert, and this is applicable to social professionals as well.

1   Level 1. Novice, starting after the initial education but without practical experience in independent work settings. The novice is dependent on learnt rules and needs guidance and rather clearly defined tasks. From the beginning the novice acts independently in not too complex contexts and should have the ability to apply the learnt rule properly.

2   Level 2. Advanced beginner, has got first practice experience and is capable of interpreting and giving meaning to characteristic aspects in comparable contexts. He or she still works under supervision and acts on learnt rules.

3   Level 3. Competent professional, with two or three years' experience as a professional worker, is capable of working with a long term strategy, and analyses processes adequately. Work is based on a deliberate planning of a

conscious, abstract, analytical contemplation of the context, and achieves efficiency.

4   Level 4. The proficient professional, has an overview, is quick in analysing and identifying the important aspects and clues and is able to compare the context with a range of comparable contexts he or she has experienced before. The proficient professional perceives situations as wholes rather than in sections.

5   Level 5. The expert, takes decisions, even without deliberate analysing and reasoning. The expert has built up an intuitive knowledge and focuses directly on the important aspects. She or he has an intuitive grasp of each situation and comes direct to action based on his or her enormous experience, knowledge and (learnt) intuition.

Social work research and social work science

The discourse

As previously mentioned, social work in itself is a knowledge-based profession. We find a huge body of knowledge on practices and methods, on policy making and on scientific disciplines integrated into social work, such as psychology, sociology, pedagogy, law, health science, public administration, ethnography. The lack of an overarching theory and recognized concept is less problematic because modern sciences are quite often currently lacking strong theoretical worldwide recognized principles and concepts. The new paradigm of science is actually recognizing the lack of paradigms or the mix of them (Kuhn 1970, Bohm and Peat 1987). To be scientific means to refer to a body of knowledge and a field of action as a discourse where complexity, research and theories are debated, analysed and constructed. The interdisciplinary character of social work should be an extra argument for recognition as a scientific field. The complexity and the variety in social work is another. The fact that complex social processes are unpredictable is no argument to exclude social work from scientific research; on the contrary. If science sticks to predictability it restricts the understanding of life to a high extent. In humanities we need room for researching and theorizing contextual realities and open processes. This approach is close to the so-called Mode 2 in current research debates (Gibbons *et al.* 1994, Nowotny *et al.* 2001). Mode 1 stands, according to those scientists, for the old science paradigm, that is to characterize as theoretical, experimental, steered by a discipline-related approach, and the autonomy of scientists and their universities. Science should be as independent as possible from daily society. Mode 2 is much more about sharing science, oriented on application and usefulness, on being trans disciplinary or even beyond existing disciplines and accountable not only to scientists and universities, but as well to the market, the public sector and the users. Mode 2 is fully embedded, connected and in interaction with society and the communities. Mode 2 research is closely related to the concept of knowledge as a productive force in modern societies. Knowledge is different from science. In knowledge orientation the field is broader and research is one of the ways to enrich knowledge. A body of knowledge replaces the concept of a disciplinary science and is open to combining scientific research with other fields of knowledge such as practice and tacit knowledge, the implicit knowledge of people based on experience. Mode 2 research is also reflective and constructive and creative (Aken 2007). However, Mode 1 (traditional science) and Mode 2 are not from a higher or lower order, nor are they excluding each other. Mode 1 and Mode 2 should be seen as complementary, to be considered as two important ways of getting knowledge and to develop sciences (Harrison and Fahy 2005). This approach is highly supported by the new universities (universities for applied science) and sometimes firmly contested and more often neglected by the old universities.

Social work research is mostly Mode 2 research, because the nature of its object of research is human beings and their mutual relationships, and the relationships between people and society. Social work scientists often prefer to speak about applied science. Applied science suggests that this science applies existing science into practice. The core seems to be the implementation and transfer of science. However, most social work research focuses on researching contexts and professional practices. It brings forward new knowledge about this specific context or specific practice. Even more than that: social sciences get the most knowledge of people and societies by researching daily life and the contexts people are in. I suggest the next research definition.

> Social work research investigates a specific context or practice in such a way that it has a recognized validity and value for all involved (financier, target group, researchers) and creates clues for improving practice and contexts. The main focus is on small scale research, action research directly aiming at improvement of practice.
>
> (Ewijk and Wilken 2005)

Important in this definition is the recognition by users and/or professionals (Marsh 2007). The perspective is on recognition and usefulness for the people involved. The role of researchers is to safeguard scientific quality (research design, research methodology and research standards).

However, social work research is not fully characterized as applied science or Mode 2 research. In fact, elements of social work are open to evidence-based research ('what works'), which is more in the field of Mode 1 research. Interesting fields of evidence-based research are identified in child care, rehabilitation and young people at risk interventions, like 'Communities that care' (Resnick and Burt 1996, Loeber and Farington 1998, Sheldon and Chilvers 2000, Luckock 2002, Konijn and Yperen 2003). In evidence-based care, researchers attempt to prove that methods and approaches in social work are to be assessed as effective or not effective. By that, social work can become more effective and will lead to a more valued and recognized profession. The-what-works debate among social work researchers is getting a lot of attention because through new management theories the 'what works' principle is claimed to be essential and is often contested by the social professionals. We should remember that the 'what works agenda' started in a period when 'nothing works' was a dominant thought, when Martinson published an article about the effects of crime prevention and recidivism (Martinson 1979). 'What works' was coined in the report to the United States Congress where scholars presented an overview on promising interventions in rehabilitation (Sherman (1996), cited in Hermans and Menger 2009). It gave a new impulse to the recognition of social work as a serious profession. The actual problem in evidence-based work with respect to generalist front line work is the fact that social workers are rarely confronted with similar situations and similar solutions. The profession is basically composed of a dynamic interactive process of interpretation, construction, implementation and evaluation in permanent different contexts. Another important consideration is the fact that evidence-based researchers are indicating that the quality of relationship between professional and user (40 per cent) and the motivation and competences of users (40 per cent) are mostly contributing to effective interventions. The applied method itself contributes approximately 15 per cent (Yperen 2004, Duncan 2006). Therefore, the room for quite expensive evidence-based research on specific methods is small, but worth continuing with, because more insight into effective methods and more understanding about what works in those methods is without doubt useful and strengthens the social professions. Overall, evidence-based research on a broader focus than methods seems more promising, taking into account the user, the professional, the specific context and the interactions. Evidence-based social work as a method originated from the education sector and started from the idea that a reflective practitioner uses the most adequate scientific knowledge, practice knowledge, personal experience and critical constructive power to decide what to do in a specific case. It is a process that is researchable and learnable. Later evidence-based research focused on research with effective methods with a strong belief in strict protocols and guidelines (Hutschemaekers and Tiemens 2006).

Different research fields

Research is to categorize in Mode 1 and Mode 2 or in description (how things are), or understanding (how it works) or in evidence (what works). In this section we look at social work focusing on four different research fields.

Professional practices research

This is mainly on the primary process, the interaction between user and professional. We can distinguish research on the process, research on satisfaction, on evaluation and effect, and on the development and design of new methods and strategies. Most of this research and development aims at specific contexts or specific fields of activities. Meta research on the findings of those researches, similarities, differences, overarching issues and findings is rare but important and creates a more intersubjective-based body of knowledge.

Contextual research

A second research domain is contextual research. A first field is investigating a social problem, a problematic situation or social source, aiming at individuals, groups or communities. Community research, as discussed in Chapter 4, covers different types of research such as social fabric, social infrastructure, contexts and demographic research. A specific field is diagnosis, intake and assessment research, as often applied in assessment agencies in youth care and long term care.

System research

I introduce the word 'system' referring to the organization and policy-making level in social policy and social work. Social work research is also about analysing functioning of social services, social policy, the interaction between users, professionals, services and the public sector and the interaction within a social service or public sector.

Trend research

The fourth domain is about trends, opinions, feelings, demographic developments, in societies and local communities and in what ways those trends affect social work practice, mostly carried out in more quantitative research designs and statistics.

Research Masters competences[1]

We conclude this chapter with an overview on research competences.

Scientific competence

COMPETENCES IN RESEARCH

- to have a critical insight into scientific literature and research in social work and social policy and to use resources adequately;
- to be able to analyse critically societal situations, problem definitions and developments and to interpret them from different theoretical frameworks and to transfer them into research designs;
- to draft a relevant, coherent and consistent research design;
- to select, apply and evaluate independently proper methods for qualitative and quantitative research;
- to select and apply analytical and constructive techniques and to be able to interpret them critically;
- to set up, carry out and evaluate research;
- to plan, manage and account for the research;
- to safeguard and guarantee its scientific quality;
- to formulate recommendations and discussions and to reflect on the research results.

- to have an advanced knowledge of social theories, social work and social policy theories and social work practice;
- to be able to integrate, conceptualize and review critically the different theories and practices;
- to analyse and apply social work and social policy-related knowledge from different disciplines, such as sociology, psychology, economy, pedagogy, anthropology and law;
- to reflect critically on complex contextual problems;
- to analyse and apply the core tasks in social work;
- to assess people's needs, contexts and behaviour;
- to be able to analyse and interpret societal problems and trends, in particular in the social domains, such as social protection and social security, housing, labour market, health, education and social services;
- to be able to analyse and interpret the functioning of social systems and their impact on human behaviour;
- to implement social policies into practice.

Intellectual and professional competence

- to have a critical, reflective and integral professional attitude, based on scientific orientation, social imagination, creative and constructive powers and independence;
- to reflect systemically and critically on one's own way of thinking, behaving and acting;
- to possess the quality, drive and attitude to be permanently active in developing knowledge, lifelong learning and managing one's own professional career;
- to contribute to the development of the discipline, the profession and the community and society;
- to innovate methods, policy-making processes and research strategies;
- to present and to profile the discipline and profession;
- to have an international orientation on theory, practice and international social policy;
- to participate in and to relate to societal debates and to value social, historical, cultural, economic and political aspects.

- to be able to communicate properly with all kinds of users, scientists, policy makers, managers, colleagues and the media;
- to be able to communicate, collaborate and manage in different contexts;
- to be able to communicate orally and in writing, about the scientific research carried out;

- to lead and to be leading in projects, researches and collaboration activities;
- to plan social processes and activities (analyse, design, plan, do, evaluate).

Discussion and assignment

Discussion

- Do you think it is important to profile and to develop social work as a field of research and as a recognized science? Why or why not?
- Do you agree or disagree with the domain and subjects of social work research? Give your reasons.

Reflection

Reflect on all the things said about professionalization and reconsider the ethical dilemmas and wonder if you feel recognized by what is said about professionalization.

Assignment

Write an essay (approximately five pages) with your reflection and your opinion on professionalization and/or social work research. It is up to you which elements you will select to reflect on.

Conclusion

Social work and social work research are exciting fields of action and science because they are about human beings, their behaviour and their relationships and about communities and societies and social cohesion and inclusion, protection and activation, on rights and obligations, on citizens in societies in transformation. I hope this book was inspiring, challenging, informing and recognizable for you. I would be very pleased to receive critical and constructive comments.

Annex
Summary of the book in keywords and definitions

This annex helps the reader to keep in mind the issues discussed in this book. For students it is a check to see if they are able to explain the keywords and definitions.

1 International social work and international social policy

Different meanings of international social work and social policy

- cross-border social work;
- comparative studies;
- advocacy;
- cross-cultural and intercultural competences and awareness;
- international transfer of social knowledge;
- the international community:
  International work stands for a common field of action and an international body of knowledge of practice and theories, its impact on national and local social work and the belonging to an international community.

Globalization

Perspectives

- economic strategy;
- compression of time and place;
- McDonaldization;
- creating a social global;
- rising global awareness and identity.

Facing new realities

- increasing global risks (environment, economic, social);
- deepening of the divide between rich and poor, between and within countries.

Regionalization

- The European Union

  - Aims

    The Union is founded on the values of respect for human dignity, freedom, democracy, equality, the rule of law and respect for human rights, including the rights of persons belonging to minorities. These values are common to the member states in a society in which pluralism, non-discrimination, tolerance, justice, solidarity and equality between women and men prevail.

  - History

    - 1951 European Coal and Steel Community;
    - 1993 European Union;
    - 2007 27 member states.

  - Structure and governance

    - European Council;
    - European Commission;
    - European Parliament;
    - European Court of Justice.

  - Some debates on the European Union

    - about governance structure and bureaucracy;
    - about civil society and civil dialogue;
    - about the EU identity and citizenship:

      Citizenship of the Union is hereby established. Every person holding the nationality of a Member State shall be a citizen of the Union.

      (Maastricht Treaty, Article 8.1)

    - about economic, environmental and social problems and their interdependence.

- The Council of Europe

  - History

    - 1949 established;
    - 1959 European Court of Human Rights;
    - 2007 47 member states.

  - Structure and governance

    - Committee of Ministers;
    - Parliamentary Assembly;
    - Congress of Local and Regional Authorities.

- The Bologna Declaration

  Adoption of a system of easily readable and comparable degrees, in order to promote European citizens' employability.

  Adoption of a system essentially based on two main cycles, undergraduate (Bachelors) and graduate (Masters). The first cycle lasts for a minimum of three years.

2 From welfare to workfare: the great transformation

From welfare to workfare

- What binds society together?
- Workfare: welfare through work.

Privatization

Why privatization is popular

- Split steering and rowing.
- Competition improves quality and effectiveness.
- Privatization decreases public expenditure and boosts the economy.
- Makes people less dependent.

The impact on social work

- introduction of personal budget;
- introduction of tendering;
- upcoming market of freelancers;
- upcoming market of small (family) businesses;
- upcoming of (multi)national firms in social welfare and social care.

Debate

- reduces public costs;
- growing market;
- more innovation and dynamic;
- more exclusion;
- fewer volunteers and informal carers;
- economizing the social;
- from social cohesion to self-interest;
- overall higher costs.

Civil society

Why civil society is popular

Civil society as representing all citizens' activities outside the public sector and market who work for the sake of the common goods and common interests.

(Naidoo 2003)

- participation as an essential factor for productive and sound societies;
- makes people less dependent on the state and public service;
- needs enough people to care for each other.

Active citizenship

- the principle of self-responsibility;
- the principle of human and social rights;
- the principle of social responsibility:
    - decent behaviour;
    - moral sensitivity;
    - commitment.

Contextual active citizenship

Citizenship is not an absolute norm (criterion) but a relative one. Each person to their own capabilities.

The impact on social work

- The Dutch case (Social Support Act)
    - guaranteeing civil rights on the local level;
    - the right to cope with your own working and living conditions;
    - the right to meet other people, the right to choose between services;
    - the right to be informed;
    - the right to complain;
    - the right to have a say;
    - the right on access.
- Debate
    - the risk of de-professionalization;
    - the risk of over-demanding vulnerable people;
    - the risk of overcharging informal carers and volunteers;
    - the risk of overcharging women.

Localization

Why localization is popular

- Social problems are contextual.
- Closer to the citizen.
- Local communities as value.
- Local communities as preventive power.
- Local communities as feeling good.

The impact on social work

- Local communities lack capacity for managing the social field.
- Local communities lack the power of decision in many cases.
- Poor municipalities create poor social services.
- Strengthens local communities.
- Creates more opportunities for integrative approaches.

Conflicting strategies

- the community strategy, based on citizen–community relationship;
- the market strategy, based on consumer–producer relationship;
- reconciling the strategies: community-based front line;
- market-based additional services.

Integration

Why integration is discussed so much

- growing mobility;
- growing diversity.

Elements

- smooth integration;
- brain drain;
- parallel societies;
- exclusion;
- illegality;
- hard criminal core;
- religious radicalism and terrorism;
- clash of civilizations.

Perspectives

- discrimination;
- normalization and assimilation;
- diversity, multicultural and intercultural perspectives;
- the multi-actor perspective.

The impact on social work

- marginal neighbourhoods, the problem of double diversities;
- integration as a threatening process;
- social work as promoting diversity and integration.

*From a macro socio-economic strategy to a micro
socio-cultural strategy*

Is the nation state losing its social interest?

- getting rid of social expenditures;
- handing the social over to the market, civil society and municipalities.

The shift to micro socio-cultural strategies

- Socio-economic quest: to combine freedom and equality.
- Work, work, work does not automatically create social cohesion.
- Opposition to the greedy individual.
- World felt as inhospitable.
- Postmodern society is highly complex and demanding.
- It is more secure in getting food, shelter, education, comfort but insecure in its relationships, communities, religions.
- Longing for a world to feel at home.
- Socio-cultural policy but based on a firm socio-economic basis.

3 Citizenship and civil society discourse

Citizenship and civil society

- From Greece and Rome, through Augustine to Locke and Montesquieu.
- Social liberalism (Dahrendorf).
- Communitarism (Walzer).
- Radical democrats (Frankfurt School).
- Postmodern: blurring ideologies.
- Confusing NGOs with market and public sector.

Perspectives on citizenship

- as status and privilege;
- legal-based citizenship;
- social citizenship;
- virtue-based citizenship (republicans);
- community-based citizenship;
- activating citizenship (and relational citizenship).

Marshall and the discourse on social citizenship

Civil, political and social rights

- Civil: rights anchored by the judicial system; personal rights on protection, freedom, etc.
- Political: right to vote and right to be politically eligible.

- Social: access to education, labour market, social security, housing, health; to guarantee basic social welfare.

Reciprocity

- Logic 1: getting back what you have paid for.
- Logic 2: compensating welfare risks (sickness, unemployment).
- Logic 3: compensating lack of income and poverty.

Legal and moral rights and duties

- Legal rights are based on laws and are enforceable.
- Moral rights are intentional and cannot be enforced.

Bottomore: formal and substantial citizenship

- Rights are no guarantee for accessibility and realization.
- Social rights hardly have meaning if they cannot be implemented.

The Ethnic perspective

- Exclusion from rights in many cases.
- Citizenship and rights seen from a different angle.

From social rights to human rights in the individualized context

- Human value in itself.

Lister: excluding and including tendency to social citizenship

Citizenship's excluding tendency

- Citizenship as a normative concept is exclusive.
- It is based on the male norm and public arena.
- Citizens' agency is performed in a variety of ways.
- We need a gender-inclusive citizenship.
- Exclusion from without (not letting in).
- Exclusion from within (being in but not accepted).

Difference and universalism

- claim for particularity;
- politics of difference;
- differentiated universalism;
    - synthesis of social rights, political participation, civic agency;
    - differences within such as gender, class, ethnicity.

Activating citizenship within the welfare state

- Bridging the gaps or undermining social citizenship.
- Participation and activation on the foreground.

Critical debates about social and activating citizenship

- Risk of exclusion by a normative approach.
- Over-demanding and overcharging.
- Tension between social, civil and political rights.
- Protection by the state, against the state and from the state.
- Who is responsible for implementing activating citizenship?
- Recognizing diversity is accepting diversity in, for example, economic status.
- Not to forget the rights and duties of the state.

4 Social work under construction

Clarifying the basics

Social work as a broad concept

- the lack of recognition;
- fragmentation;
- not defining borders, overlapping competences;
- employability;
- the Bologna Declaration;
- social professionals as family and common identity.

Different meanings of social work

- field of activities;
- professional domain or network of social professions;
- specific and specialist profession among social professions;
- body of knowledge.

Different roots

- social (case) work;
- social pedagogy;
- psychology;
- community work;
- community development;
- social care;
- socio-art therapy and community art.

Different theories

- Social work as task-centred work:
  - preventive, short interventions, methodical, problem solving.
- Constructive social work:
  - de-construction, co-construction, contextual, narrative, meaningful.
- Managerialism:
  - consumer, services/products, choice, efficiency, evidence, user rights, user involvement.
- Social pedagogy:
  - social environment, supportive, development, process, social competences.
- Critical social work:
  - macro-economic mechanisms and forces, solidarity, fighting exclusion.
- Anti-oppressive social work:
  - liberation from oppression, power over/to/of, transformative power.
- Faith-based social work:
  - spirituality, belief, meaningfulness, dignity, reconciliation, need-orientation, commitment to the poor.

The impact of the transformation

Citizenship-based social work

> The social work profession promotes social change, problem solving in human relationships, and the empowerment and liberation of people to enhance wellbeing. Utilizing theories of human behaviour and social systems, social work intervenes at the points where people interact with their environments. Principles of human rights and social justice are fundamental to social work.
>
> (IFSW and IASSW)

And

> Citizen based social work, as a field of action, knowledge and research, aims at integration of all citizens, and supports and encourages self-responsibility, social responsibility and the implementation of social rights.

The corners of social work

- reflexive therapeutic;
- socialist-collective;
- individualist-reformist;
- contextual-transformational.

Three basic postions

- front line workers;
- entrepreneurs;
- specialists.

Core tasks

- to implement social rights and duties;
- to activate people;
- to promote social cohesion;
- to strengthen social competences;
- to manage care;
- to intervene;
- to supervise and control.

Meta-methodology of social work

Explanation of basic terminology

- The professional methodology is a specified and systematic way of carrying out the professional tasks and activities that is basically recognized and recognizable for the professionals in that profession.
- A method is a specified and systematic way to achieve a defined objective.
- An instrument is a precise specified and prescriptive action to achieve a certain activity or task.

PLANNING

The methodology of social professionals

Investigating and defining the starting position (problem, request, idea).

Orientation	investigating the context of the planned action;
	investigating former experiences and actions;
	use scientific and practical knowledge.
Definition	problem, core questions, objectives.
Design	what, where, when, for whom, with whom, how, why;
	selection of methods;
	drafting a plan;
	drafting a working structure.

ACTION

Do	what is in the plan and design;
	apply the methods properly;

	use the instruments;
	be focused.
Reflect	be aware of what is happening;
	reflect and rethink.
Adjust	the method if needed;
	the attitude if needed;
	the strategy, plan and design if needed.

CONCLUSION

Evaluation	process;
	outcomes (products, results, effects);
	what has been done, why and how effective.
Accounting for	the management and financier;
	the user, participant, client;
	the process and the outcomes.
Implementation	sustainability;
	creating supporting conditions.

Co-operation and embedment

- connect to users, colleagues, managers, authorities, media;
- connect to the social fabric and the social infrastructure;
- strategic integration.

Three powers in social processes

- power of definition: user, residents (if needed supported by professionals);
- power of decision: financier;
- power of implementation: users and professionals.

Competences

A competence is the integration of knowledge, skills, attitude and reflection applied in a specific task in a certain context and contributing to an appropriate performance and result.

Competences and knowledge

- The need for exploring the main fields of knowledge.

Levels of competence

- Criteria: complexity, independence, responsibility, risks, transfer.

Assessments

- performance assessment;
- portfolio assessment;
- case analysis, problem solving;
- self- , peer, client and staff evaluation.

The competences in social work

- Primary process:

  - to communicate;
  - to assess contexts, individuals, needs, actions;
  - to plan;
  - to carry out the core tasks (see above);
  - to co-operate.

- Managerial competences:

  - to adapt to an organization;
  - to manage;
  - to develop and implement social policies.

- Professional competences:

  - to plan one's own personal career;
  - to profile and to present;
  - to innovate.

Competence-based learning

- Curriculum meets the competences.
- Didactic meets competence learning.
- Competence-based assessments.

The social professional

This professional is fully aware of living and working in a permanent transforming context. For her or him changes in (international) social policy and the diversity of residents are highly relevant.

The body of knowledge is based on the professional practice, social work theories and neighbouring scientific fields and coloured by citizenship-based social work.

5 Community policy and community work

Community-based social policy

A short history of the Western (local) community concept

- based on morality and virtue (polis);
- based on rules and power (Roman period);
- based on Civitas Dei (Christianity);
- based on utalitarianism and self-interest;
- Weber: society based on bureaucracy;
- Marx: society based on solidarity;
- Durkheim: society based on labour;
- the welfare state: based on affluence, freedom and certain level of equality;
- activating welfare state: cohesion, participation, diversity.

Re-inventing the local community

- Contextual approaches.
- Community care.
- It takes a village to raise a child.
- Safe and secure neighbourhood.
- Revitalizing neighbourhoods: the economic argument.
- Integration and diversity.
- De-institutionalization.
- Participation and civil society.

The concept of community

A local community is a small-scale territory where people live and interact based on a feeling of belonging and trust.

Community as habitat

ZONES

- social educational zone;
- social care zone;
- attractive, safe and secure community.

COMMUNITY-BASED SOCIAL POLICY

- grassroots perspective;
- educational perspective;
- capacity-building perspective;
- participation perspective;
- planning perspective;

- managing perspective;
- communitarian perspective.

The complexity of community-based social policy

- Conflicting concepts and steering strategies:

  - sector, programme, territory steering;
  - independent actors (market, national level);
  - internal bureaucracy;
  - different perceptions;
  - unclear concepts;
  - different time and scale perceptions;
  - conflicting democratic and participative principles.

Innovation from outside	*Innovation from inside*
Programming, projects	Organic improvement
Results, effects, outcomes	Gradual processes
Short term planning	Long term objectives
Managerial driven	Civil society driven
Policy makers responsible	Participative responsibility
Discontinuity	Sustainability

Promising strategies

- transparency and clarity;
- local knowledge;
- combining strategies:

  - changing the population;
  - improving the services;
  - endorsing participation;
  - improving the physical, economic and social infrastructure.

Community work

Short history

- community centres (Toynbee Hall, settlement movement);
- youth work;
- community building;
- community care.

Definition

Community work is the contribution from social professionals, together with and geared to the local citizens, in strengthening social cohesion, social capital and social competences of communities and their residents.

Social work roles, tasks and methods in community work

- To endorse and promote participation and activation:
  - informal participation;
  - volunteering and civil society;
  - labour participation;
  - democratic participation.

Social education and social cultural work

- community-building work;
- social management;
- case and care management;
- information and consultation.

Community work research and local knowledge

Local knowledge is knowledge about residents, about perceived problems, about resources to use for improving the individual and collective (community) context:

- statistical data;
- social, economic and physical infrastructure;
- social fabric, human resources, networks;
- social contexts;
- community research.

6 Other fields of activity

Youth work and youth care

Integrated sectors, bridging competencies and integrative identities

- fragmentation;
- pressure on youth care (waiting lists);
- de-concentration of residential institutes;
- children: pre-eductation or social pedagogy;
- to learn and to learn to live and live together.

To invest in young people

- protection;
- investment;
- fear and concern.

Ecologic pedagogy and integrated, contextual related approaches

- need for a strong and cohesive environment;
- need for co-operation;
- strengthening local and family networks;
- anti-institutional, user oriented.

Mapping the domain

- family support;
- child care;
- leisure time and youth work;
- youth care.

Long term care

Understanding care

- *from* protection;
- normalization;
- diversity;
- *to* co-citizenship.

Integrated care

- support: the core;
- combined actions of different actors;
- Integrated services.

Mapping the domain

- elderly care;
- care for the disabled;
- mental health care.

Social case work, exclusion and poverty

Poverty and exclusion: clarification of terms

- Relative and absolute poverty.

Different explanations for poverty and exclusion

- Society and systems are excluding.
- Exclusion by excluding inter-human mechanisms and interactions.
- Lack of competences and social capital (networks and trust).
- Disorders and disasters.

Mapping the domain

- social case work and case management;
- rehabilitation;
- shelter;
- multi-problem approach;
- integration;
- therapies.

7 From assimilation to intercultural competences: a challenge for social work

Migration and migration theories

- Economic discourse:

    - movement of low skilled migrants;
    - movement of high skilled migrants;
    - the global city (robbing the county);
    - dual market.

- Socio-cultural discourse:

    - melting pot;
    - assimilation;
    - absorption;
    - cultural pluralism;
    - multicultural and diversity.

- Transnational regionalization:

    - de-territorializes way of life;
    - multinational migrant communities;
    - world without borders.

- Diversity in Europe by migration:

    - two cases;
    - Germany;
    - Spain.

- European countries in a statistical overview.

Intercultural social work

The discourse

- interculturality as concept;
- recognition of differences and similarities in a changing contextual historic framework.

Intercultural competence

- openness to new understanding;
- communication in respecting different backgrounds;
- empathy to the other;
- multi-perspective;
- self-reflection in the perspective of difference and affinity;
- coping with insecurity and unpredictability;
- flexibility to adapt to new contexts and users;
- conflict capability to speak free from violence and to intervene properly;
- knowledge about background;
- knowledge about construction;
- knowledge about social meaning and function stereotypes and prejudices.

The importance of knowledge

- Culture is (partly) learnable.
- History, narratives, concepts, attitudes.

  Intercultural competence is: to understand the other against her or his economic, psychological and cultural background within his or her own context and to connect to the other in a proper way, recognizing and respecting differences and similarities with an explicit knowledge about the substance of cultures and ethnic diversity.

Challenging social work

- Social work theory and practice with intercultural, international and transnational perspective in the forefront.
- Social work curriculum based on interculturality.
- Improving and encouraging social work practice and practitioners to respect the intercultural perspective.
- Interculturality in social services.

8 Social work as a profession, research and science

Professionalism

Standards

- Recognizable, recognized and accepted.
- Recognized body of knowledge.
- Reflective and room for discretion:
    - conflicting interest, persons and actors;
    - to intervene or not;
    - user values and professional values;

  - involvement versus distance;
  - privacy versus public interest;
  - professional code of ethics.

- Professional code and ethics:

  - provide practitioners with guidance in their daily work;
  - make social workers trustful for the public;
  - protect users from malpractice and abuse;
  - make social professionals trustful to authorities;
  - foster a framework of understanding and professional behaviour;
  - regulate and discipline the profession;
  - protect professionals from litigation.

- Register and legal status.

Different levels

- Levels of workforce positions:

  - assistants;
  - skilled workers;
  - professional generalists;
  - specialists;
  - scientists.

- Levels of functioning:

  - novice;
  - advanced beginner;
  - competent professional;
  - proficient professional;
  - Expert.

Social work research and social work science

Discourse

- Lack of overarching theory or framework.
- Science as complex body of knowledge, without paradigm.
- Humanities: unpredictable human behaviour and relationships.
- Mode 2: sharing, application, knowledge, transdisciplinary, accountable, reflective, constructive:

Social work research investigates a specific context or practice in such a way that it has a recognized validity and value for all involved (financier, target group, researchers) and creates suggestions for improving practice and contexts. The main focus is on small-scale research, action research directly aiming at improvement of practice.

- Evidence-based research on methods.
- Evidence based on the context: user, professional, method (user 40 per cent, relationship user–professional 40 per cent, method 15 per cent).
- Evidence-based research as reflective practice: using most adequate scientific knowledge, practice knowledge, personal experiences and critical constructive power.

Different research fields

- professional practice;
- contexts (individual, group, network, community);
- systems (organizations, chains, policy-making process);
- trends (societal, local, neighbourhood, history and future).

Research Masters competences

- Research competences:
  - critical insight in scientific literature and research;
  - to analyse critically social contexts;
  - to draft a research design;
  - to select and apply methods;
  - to select and apply techniques;
  - to set up, carry out and evaluate research;
  - to plan, manage and account for the research;
  - to safeguard and guarantee its scientific quality;
  - to recommend, discuss and reflect on research results.

- Competence in social work and social policy theory and practice:
  - advanced knowledge of social theories, social policy, social work theories and social work practice;
  - to overview, review and integrate theories and practices;
  - to analyse and apply social work/policy-related theories;
  - to analyse and apply the core tasks in social work/policy;
  - to assess people's needs, contexts and behaviour;
  - to reflect critically on complex social work contexts;
  - to analyse and interpret societal problems and trends;
  - to analyse the functioning and impact of social systems;
  - to implement social policies into practice.

- Competences in professionalization:
  - critical, reflective and integral, scientific, constructive;
  - to reflect critically on personal functioning;
  - drive to livelong learning;
  - to contribute to the discipline and profession;

- to innovate methods, strategies and processes;
- to present and to profile the discipline and profession.

Social work and social work research are exciting fields of action and science because they are about human beings, their behaviour and their relationships, and about communities and societies and social cohesion and inclusion, protection and activation, on rights and obligations, of citizens in societies in transformation.

Notes

1 International social work and international social policy

1 This chapter is (partly) an elaboration (and some parts are copied) of an article published by the author: Ewijk, H. van, 2009. Citizenship-based social work. *International Social Work*, 52, 2, 158–70.

3 Citizenship and civil society discourse

1 This is concluded in an international comparative study of the development of social duties in 18 countries, during the period 1930 to 1990. The study is based on data from a series of time in the database SCIP (Social Citizenship Indicators Project).

4 Social work under construction

1 This section is based on the author's practical experience and a range of publications, in particular: Ewijk 1985, Kloppenburg *et al.* 1991, Stepney and Ford 2000, Schilling 2008.
2 This section is based on the internal competence schemes of Hogeschool Utrecht, Universiteit van Gent and Tartu Ülikool, and scientific resources such as Ashworth and Saxton 1990, Hager and Gonczi 1991, Tesluk and Jacobs 1998, Nedermeijer and Pilot 2000.

6 Other fields of activity

1 Ecologic pedagogy is used in two different senses. First, it refers to social education in environmental awareness, and second, it refers to a pedagogy integration of micro, meso and macro systems.

7 From assimilation to intercultural competences: a challenge for social work

1 This section is mainly based on Petrus Hans study and overview of migrant theories (Han 2007).
2 Translation: The absolute multicultural hypothesis is absurd as the cultural homogeneity of a city or a country. Intercultural relations are the only reality.

8 Social work as a profession, research and science

1 Inspired by competence schemes of the Universiteit van Gent and Tartu Ülikool.

Bibliography

Adams, R., Dominelli, L. and Payne, M., eds. 2002. *Social work: themes, issues and critical debates*, 2nd edn. Basingstoke: Palgrave.

Ahmadi, N. 2003. Globalization of consciousness and new challenges for international social work. *International Journal of Social Welfare*, 12 (1), 14–23.

Aken, J.E. van. 2007. *Organization studies as applied science: finding firm ground in the swamp* (research paper). Eindhoven: University of Technology.

Alcock, P., Glennerster, H., Oakley A., and Sinfield A., eds. 2001. *Welfare and wellbeing: Richard Titmuss's contribution to social policy*. Bristol: The Policy Press.

Ålund, A. 2002. Sociala problem i kulturell förklädnad. In A. Meeuwisse and H. Swärd, eds, *Perspektiv på sociala problem*. Stockholm: Natur och Kultur, 293–31.

Ålund. A. 2005. Etnicitet, medborgarskap och gränser. In P. de los Reyes, I. Molina and D. Mulinari, eds, *Maktens (o)lika förklädnader Kön, klass & etnicitet i det postkoloniala Sverige*. Stockholm: Bokförlaget Atlas, 285–94.

Ashworth, P.D. and Saxton, J. 1990. On competence. *Journal of Further and Higher Education*, 14, 2, 3–25.

Ayaan, H. 2006. *The caged virgin: an emancipation proclamation for women and Islam*. London: Simon & Schuster.

Bahmüller, C. 2002. Civil society and democracy. In NIZW, *Bridging the gaps: essays on economic, social and cultural opportunities at global and local levels*. Utrecht: NIZW, 71–9.

Baldock, J., Manning, N. and Vickerstaff, S., eds. 2003. *Social policy*, 2nd edn. Oxford: Oxford University Press.

Banks, J. and Banks, C. eds, 1989. *Multicultural education: issues and perspectives*. Boston: Allyn and Bacon.

Banks, S. 2006. *Ethics and values in social work*, 3d edn. Basingstoke: BASW, Palgrave.

Barbuto, D.M. 1999. *The American settlement movement: a bibliography*. Westport: Greenwood Press.

Barnes, C., Oliver, M. and Barton, L. 2002. *Disability studies today*. Cambridge: Polity Press.

Bauböck, R. and Rundell, J., eds. 1998. *Blurred boundaries: migration, ethnicity, citizenship*. Aldershot, Brookfield, Singapore and Sydney: Ashgate.

Bauman, Z. 2001. *Community: seeking safety in an insecure world*. Oxford and Malden: Polity Press.

Beck, U. 1986. *Risikogesellschaft: auf dem Wege in eine andere Moderne*. Frankfurt am Main: Suhrkamp.

Benner, P. 1984. *From novice to expert: excellence and power in clinical nursing practice*. Menlo Park: Addison-Wesley.

Berkel, R. van and Møller, H. 2002. The concept of activation. In R. van Berkel and H. Møller, eds, *Active social policies in the EU: inclusion through participation?* Bristol: The Policy Press, 45–71.

Berkel, R. van, Møller, H. and Williams, C.C. 2002. The concept of inclusion/exclusion and the concept of work. In R. van Berkel and H. Møller, eds, *Active social policies in the EU: inclusion through participation?* Bristol: The Policy Press, 15–44.

Bie, M. de and Ewijk, H. van, eds. 2008. *Sociaal werk in Nederland en Vlaanderen: een begrippenkader.* Mechelen: Kluwer.

Bohm, D. and Peat, F.D. 1987. *Science, order, and creativity.* New York: Bantam Books.

Bologna Declaration. 1999. *The Bologna Declaration on the European space for higher education: an explanation.* www.ec.europa.eu/education/policies/educ/bologna/bologna.pdf (accessed 17 January 2009).

Bottomore, T. 1992. *Citizenship and social class.* London: Pluto Press.

Bourdieu, P. 1984. *Distinction, a social critique of the judgement of taste.* Cambridge, MA: Harvard University Press.

Bourdieu, P. and Passeron, J.C. 1970. *La reproduction, éléments pour une théorie du système d'enseignement.* Paris: Les éditions de minuit.

Boutellier, H. 2002. *De veiligheidsutopie: hedendaags onbehagen en verlangen rond misdaad en straf.* Den Haag: Boom Juridische Uitgevers.

Bouverne-de Bie, M. and Ewijk, H. van. 2008. Een inleiding aan de hand van een aantal kernbegrippen. In M. de Bie and H. van Ewijk, eds, *Sociaal werk in Nederland en Vlaanderen: een begrippenkader.* Mechelen: Kluwer, 17–56.

Brink, B. van der. 1994. De civil society als 'kloppend' hart van de maatschappij: drie filosofische visies. In P. Dekker, ed., *Civil society: civil society en vrijwilligerswerk I.* Den Haag: SCP, 49–66.

Bronfenbrenner, U. 1979. *The ecology of human development: experiment by nature and design.* Cambridge, MA: Harvard University Press.

Bronfenbrenner, U. 1986. Ecology of the family as a context for human development. *Developmental Psychology*, 22, 723–42.

Cambridge, P. and Ernst. A. 2006. Comparing local and national service systems in social care Europe: framework and findings from the STEPS anti-discrimination learning disability project. *European Journal of Social Work*, 9, 3, 279–303.

Cameron, C. and Moss, P. 2007. *Care work in Europe: current understandings and future directions.* London and New York: Routledge.

Canda, E.R. 1998. Afterword: linking spirituality and social work: five themes for innovation. In E.R. Canda, ed., *Spirituality in social work: new directions.* New York: Haworth Press, 97–106.

Cannan, C. and Warren, C. eds. 1997. *Social action with children and families: a community development approach to child and family welfare.* London: Routledge.

Castells, M. 1999. *The informational city: information technology, economic restructuring and the urban-regional process.* Oxford and Malden, MA: Blackwell Publishers (first published 1989).

Chanan, G. 1997. *Active citizenship and community involvement: getting to the roots.* Luxembourg: Office for Official Publications of the European Union.

Clinton, H.C. 1996. *It takes a village.* New York: Simon & Schuster.

Comité des Sages. 1996. *For a Europe of civic and social rights: report by the Comité des Sages.* Luxembourg: Office for Official Publications of the European Communities.

Communities that care (CTC). 2008. http://www.communitiesthatcare.org.uk/ (accessed 13 December 2008).

Council of Europe. 2001. *Report of the Educational Council to the European Council. The concrete future objectives of education and training systems.* 5680/01, EDUC 18.

Council of Europe. 2009a. http://www.coe.int/T/e/Com/about_coe/ (accessed 13 January 2009).

Council of Europe. 2009b. http://www.coe.int/T/E/Com/About_Coe/DiscoursChurchill.asp (accessed 13 January 2009).

Cox, R.H. 1998. The consequences of welfare reform: how conceptions of social rights are changing, *Journal of Social Policy*, 27, 1–16.

Cree, V.E. 2002. The changing nature of social work. In R. Adams, L. Dominelli and M. Payne, *Social work: themes, issues and critical debates*. Basingstoke: Palgrave, pp 20–9.

Crockett, L.J. and Crouter, A.C. eds. 1995. *Pathways through adolescence: individual development in social contexts*. Mahwah, NJ: L. Erlbaum Associates, 211–33.

Dahl, R.A. 1998. *On democracy*. New Haven and London: Yale University Press.

Dahrendorf, R. 1988. *The modern social conflict*. New York: Weidenfeld & Nicolson, 34–5.

Deacon, B. 2000. *Globalization and social policy*. Geneva: UN.

Deacon, B., Ollila, E., Koivusalo, M. and Stubbs, P. 2003. *Global social governance: themes and prospects*. Helsinki: Hakapaino Oy.

Deppe-Wolfinger, H. 1973. *Arbeiterjugend. Bewusstsein und politische Bildung*. Frankfurt am Main: Athenäum.

Deutscher Verein für öffentliche und private Fürsorge ISS, Bundesministerium für Familie, Senioren, Frauen und Jugend (DV). 2001. *Daseinsvorsorge in Europa heute und morgen – die Zukunft der kommunalen und freigemeinnützigen sozialen Dienste*. Frankfurt am Main: DV.

Doel, M. 2002. Task-centered work. In R. Adams, L. Dominelli and M. Payne, eds, *Social work: themes, issues and critical debates*. Basingstoke: Palgrave, 191–9.

Dominelli, L. 2002a. *Anti-oppressive social work: theory and practice*. Basingstoke: Palgrave Macmillan.

Dominelli, L. 2002b. Anti-oppressive practice in context. In R. Adams, L. Dominelli and M. Payne, eds, *Social work: themes, issues and critical debates*. Basingstoke: Palgrave, 3–19.

Dominelli, L. 2004. *Social work: theory and practice for a changing profession*. Malden, MA: Polity Press.

Donovan, E.J. and Walsh, W.F. 1989. Private security and community policing: evaluation and comment. *Journal of Criminal Justice*, 17, 3.

Dubois, B. and Krogsrud, M. 1999. *Social work: an empowering profession*, 3d edn. Boston: Allyn and Bacon.

Duncan, B.L. 2006. Common factors and uncommon heroism of youth. In *Congresboek jeugdzorg in onderzoek*. Utrecht: NJI.

Dunne, T. 2008. Good citizen Europe. *International Affairs*, 84, 1, 13–28.

Durkheim, E. 1986. *De la division du travail social*, 11th edn. Paris: Quadrige/Presses Universitaires de France (1st edn 1930).

Duyvendak, J.W., Knijn, T. and Kremer, M. 2006. *Policy, people, and the new professional: de-professionalisation and re-professionalisation in care and welfare*. Amsterdam: Amsterdam University Press.

East, L. 2002. Regenerating health in communities: voices from the inner city. *Critical Social Policy*, 22, 2, 147–73.

Eblen, R.A. and Eblen, W. 1994. *The encyclopedia of the environment*. Boston: Houghton Mifflin Company.

Eijken, J. van and Ewijk, H. van, eds. 2005. *Re-inventing social work*. Utrecht: Hogeschool van Utrecht.

Eisenstadt, S.N. 1954. *The absorption of immigrants: a comparative study based mainly on the Jewish community in Palestine and the State of Israel*. London: Routledge & Kegan Paul.

Ellison, N. and Pierson, C. 2003. *Developments in British social policy 2*. Basingstoke: Palgrave Macmillan.

Engberse, G., Snel, E. and Boom, J. de. 2007. *De adoptie van wijken: een evaluatie van 'Nieuwe coalities voor de Wijk'*. Rotterdam: Erasmus Universiteit/RISB.

ENSACT. *European Network for Social Action*. 2009. http://www.ensact.eu/ (accessed 24 February 2009).

Erasmus, J. 2000. *Religion and social transformation: a case study from South Africa*. Cape Town: URDR.

Erickson, P. 1992. What multiculturalism means. *Transition*, 55, 105–14.

Etzioni, A. 1993. *The spirit of community*. New York: Crown Books.

Etzioni, A., ed. 1998. *The essential communitarian reader*. Lanham, Boulder, New York, and Oxford: Rowman & Littlefield.

Etzioni, A. 2001. The third way to a good society. *Sociale Wetenschappen*, 3, 5–41.

European Commission. 1999. *A concerted strategy for modernizing social protection*. Com (1999), 347.

European Commission. 2004a. *Facing the challenge: the Lisbon strategy for growth and employment*. ISBN 92-894-7054-2 (http://ec.europa.eu/growthandjobs/index_en.htm) (High Level Group chaired by Wim Kok) (accessed 13 December 2008).

European Commission. 2004b. *Report of the high level group on the future of social policy in an enlarged European Union*. Directorate-General for Employment, Industrial Relations and Social Affairs. (http://ec.europa.eu/employment_social/news/2004/jun/hlg_social_elarg_en.pdf) (accessed 13 December 2008).

European Commission. 2005a. *Communication to the spring European Council. Working together for growth and jobs: a new start for the Lisbon Strategy*. Communication from President Barroso. com 24.

European Commission. 2005b. *Reconciliation of work and private life: a comparative review of thirty European countries*. Luxembourg: Office for Official Publications of the European Communities.

European Commission. 2006a. *Implementing the community Lisbon program: social services of general interest in the European Union*. Brussels: Com (2006), 177.

European Commission. 2006b. *Directive on services in the internal market*. 2006/123/EC.

European Union. 2009. http://europa.eu/abc/panorama/index_en.htm. (accessed 12 January 2009).

Eurostat. 2008. *Statistics in focus*. 98/2005. http://epp.eurostat.ec.europa.eu/cache/ITY_OFFPUB/KS-SF-08-098/EN/KS-SF-08-098-EN.PDF (accessed: 8 March 2009).

Evans, M. and Cerny, P. 2003. Globalization and social policy. In N. Ellison and C. Pierson, eds, *Developments in British social policy 2*. Basingstoke: Palgrave Macmillan, 19–40.

Ewijk, H. van. 1985. *Methodiek in het jeugdwerk*. Alphen a.d. Rijn: Samson.

Ewijk, H. van. 2006. Changing diversity in social work. *European Journal of Social Education*, 10/11, 31–45.

Ewijk, H. van. 2007. Integration and transformation: the need for a citizenship-based social work. *European Journal of Social Education*, 12/13, 15–26.

Ewijk, H. van. 2008a. Actief Burgerschap. In V. de Waal, ed., *Samenspel in de buurt: burgers, sociale professionals en beleidsmakers aan zet.* Utrecht: SWP, 19–34.

Ewijk, H. van. 2008b. Burgers en buurten. In V. de Waal, ed., *Samenspel in de buurt: burgers, sociale professionals en beleidsmakers aan zet.* Utrecht: SWP, 99–113.

Ewijk, H. van. 2009. Citizenship-based social work. *International Social Work*, 52 (2), 158–70.

Ewijk, H. van and Wilken, J.P. 2005. Developing research practices in social work: a challenging endeavour for the Centre of Expertise for Social Policy and Social Care. In J. van Eijken and H. van Ewijk, eds, *Re-inventing social policy.* Utrecht: HU, 115–23.

Ewijk, H. van, Spierings, F. and Wijnen, R., eds. 2007. *Basisboek social work: mensen en meedoen.* Amsterdam: Boom.

Ewijk, H. van, Hens, H., Lammersen G. and Moss, P. eds. 2002. *Care work in Europe, workpackage 4, mapping of care services and the care workforce. Consolidated report.* London: Thomas Coram Institute, London University.

Federal Statistical Office Germany. http://www.destatis.de/jetspeed/portal/cms/Sites/destatis/Internet/EN/Navigation/Homepage__NT.psml (accessed 9 March 2009).

Ferguson, K.M. 2005. Beyond indigenization and reconceptualization. Towards a global, multidirectional model of technology transfer. *International Social Work*, 48, 5, 519–35.

Ferguson, R.F. and Dickens, W.T., eds. 1999. *Urban problems and community development.* Washington: Brookings Institution Press.

Freise, J. 2005. *Interkulturelle Soziale Arbeit. Theoretische Grundlagen – Handlungsansätze – Übungen zum Erwerb interkultureller Kompetenz.* Schwalbach: Wochenschau Verlag.

Gaitanides, S. 2003. Interkulturelle Kompetenz als Anforderungsprofil in der Jugend- und Sozialarbeit. *Sozialmagazin*, 3, 42–8.

Germain, C.B. and Gitterman, A. 1980. *The life model of social work practice.* New York: Columbia University Press.

Gibbons, M.C., Scott, P., Schwartzman, S., and Nowotny H., 1994. *The new production of knowledge: the dynamics of science and research in contemporary societies.* London: Sage.

Giddens, A. 1991. *Modernity and self-identity: self and society in the late modern age.* Cambridge: Polity Press.

Giddens, A. 1998. *The third way: the renewal of social democracy.* Cambridge: Polity Press.

Giddens, A. 2007. *Europe in the global age.* Malden, MA: Polity Press.

Gordon, M.M. 1964. *Assimilation in American life. The role of race, religion, and national origin.* New York: Oxford University Press.

Gunsteren, H.R. van. 1992. *Eigentijds burgerschap.* 's Gravenhage: WRR/SDU.

Gutiérrez, L., Zuñiga, M. and Lum, D. 2005. *Education for multicultural social work practice.* Alexandria: CSWE.

Hager, P. and Gonczi, A. 1991. What is competence? *Medial Teacher*, 18 (1), 15–18.

Hammar, T. 1990. *Democracy and the nation-state: aliens, denizens and citizens in a world of international migration.* Aldershot: Avebury.

Han, P. 2007. *Theorien zur internationalen Migration. Ausgewählte interdisziplinäre Migrationstheorien und deren zentralen Aussagen.* Stuttgart: Lucius and Lucius.

Handschuck, S. and Kalwe, W. 2004. *Interkulturelle Verständigung in der Sozialen Arbeit. Ein Erfahrungs-, Lern- und Übungsprogramm zum Erwerb interkultureller Kompetenz.* München: IQM.

Hansen, H.K. and Jensen, J.J. 2004. *Care work in Europe, workpackage eight: work with adults with severe disabilities. A case study of Denmark, the Netherlands and Sweden.* London: Thomas Coram Institute, London University.

Hardcastle, D.A. and Powers, P.R. 2004. *Community practice: theories and skills for social workers*, 2nd edn. New York: Oxford University Press.

Hare, I. 2004. Defining social work for the 21st century: the International Federation of Social Workers' revised definition of social work. *International Social Work*, 47, 3, 407–24.

Harrison, K. and Fahy, K. 2005. Constructive research: methodology and practice. In G.M. Tenenbaum and G.M. Driscoll, eds, *Methods of research in sports science: quantitative and qualitative approaches*. Oxford: Meyer and Meyer, 660–700.

Hayes, D. 2006. *History and context: the impact of immigration control on welfare delivery*. In D. Hayes and B. Humphries, *Social work, immigration and asylum: debates, dilemmas and ethical issues for social work and social care practice*. London and Philadelphia: Jessica Kingsley Publishers, 11–28.

Hayes, D. and Humphries, B. 2006. *Social work, immigration and asylum: debates, dilemmas and ethical issues for social work and social care practice*. London and Philadelphia: Jessica Kingsley Publishers.

Healy, L. 2001. *International social work: professional action in an interdependent world*. Oxford and New York: Oxford University Press.

Hermans, J. and Menger, A. 2009. *Walk the line*. Amsterdam: SWP.

Herz, D. and Jetzlsperger, C. 2008. *Die Europäische Union*. München: C.H. Beck.

Holden, C. 2005. Organizing across borders: profit and quality in internationalized providers. *International Social Work*, 48, 5, 643–53.

Hoskins, B.J. and Jesinghaus, I. 2006. *Measuring active citizenship in Europe: institute for the protection and security of citizens*. Eur/2530/en.

Hughes, R. 1987. *The fatal shore*. London: Collins Harvill.

Humphries, B. 2006. *The construction and reconstruction of social work*. In D. Hayes and B. Humphries, *Social work, immigration and asylum: debates, dilemmas and ethical issues for social work and social care practice*. London and Philadelphia: Jessica Kingsley Publishers, 29–42.

Huntington, S. 1997. *Botsende beschavingen: Cultuur en conflict in de 21ste eeuw*. Antwerpen: Anthos/Mantau.

Hutschemaekers, G. and Tiemens, B. 2006. Evidence-based policy: from answer to question. In J.W. Duyvendak, T. Knijn and M. Kremer, *Policy, people, and the new professional: de-professionalisation and re-professionalisation in care and welfare*. Amsterdam: Amsterdam University Press, 34–47.

Ife, J. and Fiske, L. 2006. Human rights and community work: complementary theories and practices. *International Social Work*, 49, 3, 297–308.

International Council on Social Welfare. 2006. *Review of the first UN decade for the eradication of poverty 1997–2006: one decade has passed, another to go*. Utrecht: ICSW (http://www.icsw.org/doc/2006%20UN%20ICSW%20Statement%20CSocD%20ENG.doc) (accessed 25 February 2009).

International Federation of Social Workers. 2009a. *Definition of social work*. http://www.ifsw.org/en/p38000208.html (accessed 25 February 2009).

International Federation of Social Workers. 2009b. *Ethics in social work, statement of principles*. http://www.ifsw.org/en/p38000324.html (accessed 25 February 2009).

International Federation of Social Workers. 2009c. http://www.ifsw.org/en/p38000605.html (accessed 25 February 2009).

Irving, Z. and Payne, M. 2005. Globalization: implications for teaching and learning. In H. Burgess and I. Taylor, eds, *Effective learning and teaching in social policy and social work*. London: Routledge Falmer.

Jacobs, J. 1992. *The death and life of great American cities*. New York: Vintage (originally published 1961).

Jones, C. 2002. Social work and society. In R. Adams, L. Dominelli and M. Payne, eds, *Social work: themes, issues and critical debates*. Basingstoke: Palgrave, 4–49.

Jones, D. and Mayo, M. eds. 1974. *Community work one*. London: Routledge & Kegan Paul.

Keller, S. 2003. *Community: pursuing the dream, living the reality*. Princeton: Princeton University Press.

Keller, V. 2005. *Aider et contrôler: les controverses du travail social*. Lausanne: EESP.

Khagram, S. and Levitt, P. 2008. Constructing transnational studies. In S. Khagram and P. Levitt, eds, *The transnational studies reader. Intersections and innovations*. New York and London: Routledge, 1–18.

Kloppenburg, R., Heemelaar, M., Jansen, M. and Brinkman, F. 1991. *Methodiek sociaal pedagogische hulpverlening*. Houten: Bohn, Stafleu, Van Loghum.

Knijn, T. and Kremer, M. 1997. Gender and the caring dimension of welfare states: toward inclusive citizenship. *Social Politics*, 4, 3, 328–61.

Konijn, C. and Yperen, T.A. van. 2003. *Internationaal overzicht effectieve interventies in de jeugdzorg*. Utrecht: NIZW.

Kortram, L. 2004. *Multicultureel samen(-)leven*. Zeist: De Horst.

Kröger, T. 2001. *Comparative research on social care: the state of the art*. Brussels: Soccare.

Kuhn, T.S. 1970. *The structure of scientific revolutions*, 2nd edn. Chicago: University of Chicago Press.

Lane, R.E. 2000. *The loss of happiness in market democracies*. New Haven: Yale University Press.

Lawy, R. and Biesta, G. 2006. Citizenship-as-practice: the educational implication of an inclusive and relational understanding of citizenship. *British Journal of Educational Studies*, 54, 1, 34–50.

Lipsky, M. 1980. *Street-level bureaucracy: dilemmas of the individual in public services*. New York: Russell Sage Foundation

Lisbon European Council. 2000. *Presidency conclusions*. 100/1/00.

Lister, R. 1997. Citizenship: towards a feminist synthesis. *Feminist Review*, 57, 28–48.

Lister, R. 2003. *Citizenship feminist perspectives*. New York: New York University Press.

Lister, R. 2006. Inclusive citizenship: realizing the potential. *Citizenship studies*, 11, 1, 49–61 (http://hdl.handle.net/2134/2524).

Lister, R. 2007. Inclusive citizenship: realizing the potential. *Citizenship Studies*, 11, 49–61.

Locke, J. 1689 [1990]. *An essay concerning the true, original, extent and end of civil government*. London: Dent.

Loeber, R. and Farington, D.P. 1998. *Serious and violent juvenile offenders: risk factors and successful interventions*. Thousand Oaks, CA: Sage.

Lorenz, W. 2004. *Towards a European paradigm of social work. Studies in the history of modes of social work and social policy in Europe*. Dresden: Technischen Universität.

Lorenz, W. 2006. *Perspectives on European social work – from the birth of the nation state to the impact of globalization*. Opladen: Barbara Budrich Publishers.

Luckock, B. 2002. Effective interventions for child abuse and neglect: an evidence-based approach to planning and evaluating interventions. *Child and Family Social Work*, 71, 68–89.

Lyons, K. 1999. *International social work: themes and perspectives*. Aldershot: Ashgate.

Lyons, K., Manion, K. and Carlsen, M. 2006. *International perspectives on social work. Global conditions and local practice*. Basingstoke: Palgrave Macmillan.

Maas, A. van der, Scheijmans, I. and Ewijk, H. van. 2008. *De zwanenvechtpleinbuurt*. Utrecht: HU.

Maastricht Treaty. 1972. *The Maastricht Treaty: provisions amending the treaty, establishing the European Economic Community with a view to establishing the European community*. http://www.eurotreaties.com/maastrichtec.pdf (accessed 15 February 2009).

Marcuse, H. 1964. *One dimensional man: studies in the ideology of advanced industrial society*. Boston: Beacon Press.

Marsh, P. 2007. *Developing an enquiring social work practice: practitioners, researchers and users as scientific partners*. Houten: Bohn Stafleu van Loghum, and Marie Kamphuis Stichting.

Marshall, T.H. 1950. *Citizenship and social class and other essays*. Cambridge: Cambridge University Press.

Marshall, T.H. and Bottomore, T. 1992. *Citizenship and social class*. London: Pluto Classic.

Marsland, D. 1996. *Welfare or welfare state? Contradictions and dilemmas in social policy*. Basingstoke: Macmillan Press.

Martinson, R. 1979. New findings, new views. A note of caution regarding sentencing reform. *Public Interest*, 35, 22–54.

Mkandawire, T. 2005. *Targeting und universalism in poverty reduction*. New York: United Nations.

Mkandawire, T. and Rodríguez, V. 2000. *Globalization and social development after Copenhagen: premises, promises and policies*. Geneva: UNRISD.

Monivas, A. and Ciot, M.G. 2008. Romanian migration to Spain. An intercultural approach. In G. Franger and M. Necasovsa, eds, *On the move. European social work responses to migration*. Rome: Carocci, 56–67.

Morin, E. 1988. *Penser l'Europe*. Paris: Gallimard.

Naidoo, K. 2003. *Kumi Naidoo on civil society*. www.abc.net.au (accessed 14 Dezember 2008).

National Institute for Social Work. 1982. *Social workers, their role and tasks* (The Barclay Report). London: Bedford Square Press.

Nedermeijer, J. and Pilot, A. 2000. *Beroepscompetenties en academische vorming in het hoger onderwijs*. Groningen: Wolters Noordhoff.

Neil, S. 2002. 'E-stablishing' an inclusive society? Technology, social exclusion and UK government policy making. *Journal of Social Policy*, 31, 1, 1–21.

Niemeyer, C. 2002. Sozialpädagogik, Sozialarbeit, Soziale Arbeit – 'klassische' Aspekte der Theoriegeschichte. In W. Thole, ed., *Grundriss Soziale Arbeit. Ein einführendes Handbuch*. Opladen: Leske and Budrich, 123–37.

Nimako, K. 2002. Repositioning social policy: north–south dialogue in the context of the donor–recipient relation. In NIZW, *Bridging the gaps: essays on economic, social and cultural opportunities at global and local levels*. Utrecht: NIZW, 23–34.

Nowak, J. 2001. *Netzwerk Europa. Einheit in der Vielfalt. Historische, gesellschaftliche und sprachliche Zusammenhänge sowie Lexikon der Vielfalt Europas*. Berlin: Hitit Verlag.

Nowak, J. 2006. *Leitkultur und Parallelgesellschaft. Argumente wider einen politschen Mythos*. Frankfurt am Main: Brandes und Apsel.

Nowotny, H. 2006. Real science is excellent science: how to interpret post academic science. Mode 2 and the ERC. *Journal of Science Communication*, 5, 4, 1–3.

Nowotny, H., Scott, P. and Gibbons, M. 1991. *Re-thinking science: knowledge and the public in an age of uncertainty*. Cambridge: Polity Press.

Organisation for Economic Co-operation and Development (OECD). 1999. *A caring world.* Paris: OECD.

Organisation for Economic Co-operation and Development (OECD). 2009. *Statistics portal.* http://www.oecd.org/statsportal/0,3352,en_2825_293564_1_1_1_1_1,00.html (accessed 9 March 2009).

Osborne, D. and Gaebler, T. 1992. *Reinventing government : how the entrepreneurial spirit is transforming the public sector.* Reading, MA: Addison-Wesley.

Parton, N. 1996. *Social theory, social change and social work.* London: Routledge.

Parton, N. 2002. Post modern and constructionist approaches to social work. In R. Adams, L. Dominelli and M. Payne, eds, *Social work: themes, issues and critical debates.* Basingstoke: Palgrave, 237–46.

Parton, N., O'Byrne, P. and Nijnatten, C. van. 2007. *Social work, een constructieve benadering.* Houten: Bohn, Staffleu, van Lochum.

Payne, M. 2002. Social work theories and reflective practice. In R. Adams, L. Dominelli and M. Payne, eds, *Social work: themes, issues and critical debates.* Basingstoke: Palgrave, 123–38.

Payne, M. 2005. *Modern social work theory*, 3rd edn. Basingstoke: Palgrave Macmillan.

Payne, M. 2006. *What is professional social work?* Birmingham: The Polity Press.

Pitkänen, P. 2007. Intercultural competence in work: a case study in Eastern Finnish enterprises. *Managing Global Transitions*, 54, 391–408.

Price, V. and Simpson, G. 2007. *Transforming society? Social work and sociology.* Bristol: The Policy Press.

Putnam, R.D. 1993. *Making democracy work: civic traditions in modern Italy.* Princeton: Princeton University Press.

Putnam, R.D. 2000. *Bowling alone: the collapse and revival of American community.* New York: Simon & Schuster.

Ramakers, C. and Wijngaart, M. van den. 2005. *Persoonsgebonden budget en mantelzorg. Onderzoek naar de aard en omvang van de betaalde en onbetaalde mantelzorg.* Nijmegen: ITS.

Regan, S. 2007. *Role of community work in community building*, http://www.cnm.tcd.ie/publications/workers.pdf (accessed 19 February 2009).

Resnick, G. and Burt, M.R. 1996. Youth at risk: definitions and implications for service delivery. *American Journal of Orthopsychiatry*, 66, 172–88.

Room, G. ed. 1995. *Beyond the threshold: the measurement and analysis of social exclusion.* Bristol: The Policy Press,

Sanchez, T.W., Lang, R.E. and Dhavale, D.M. 2005. Security versus status? A first look at the census; gated community data. *Journal of Planning Education and Research*, 24, 281–91.

Sassen, S. 1991. *The global city.* New York: Princeton University Press.

Scheffer, P. 2007. *Het land van aankomst.* Amsterdam: De Bezige Bij.

Scherer, A. 2002. Sozialarbeitswissenschaft. Anmerkungen zu den Grundzügen eines theoretishcen Programms. In W. Thole, ed., *Grundriss Soziale Arbeit. Ein einführendes Handbuch.* Opladen: Leske und Budrich, 259–71.

Schierup, C-U. 2003. Social exkludering och medborgarskap i Sverige och EU. In P. Blomqvist, ed., *Den gränslösa välfärdsstaten Svensk socialpolitik i det nya Europa.* Stockholm: Agora, 176–99.

Schierup, C-U. 2005. Vart tog den sociala dimensionen vägen? Medborgarskap, multikulturalism och social exkludering. In P. de los Reyes, I. Molina and D. Mulinari, eds, *Maktens (o)lika förklädnader Kön, klass ed etnicitet i det postkoloniala Sverige.* Stockholm: Bokförlaget Atlas, 237–62.

Schilling, J. 2008. *Soziale Arbeit. Geschichte, Theorie, Profession*, 3rd edn. Stuttgart: UTB.

Sennett, R. 1977 [2002]. *The fall of public man.* New York: Knopf Inc. London: Penguin Books.

Sheldon, B. and Chilvers, R. 2000. *Evidence-based social care: a study of prospects and problems.* Lyme Regis: Russell House Publishing.

Sherman, L.W., Gottfredson, D. Mackenzie, D., Eck J., Reuter P., and Bushway S., 1996. Preventing crime, what works, what doesn't and what's promising? Report to the United States Congress.

Sjöberg, O. 1999. *Paying for social rights.* Stockholm: Institutet för social forskning.

Skinner, S. 1997. *Building community strengths: a resource book on capacity building.* London: Community Development Foundation.

Smith, D. 2002. Social work with defenders. In R. Adams, L. Dominelli and M. Payne, eds, *Social work: themes, issues and critical debates.* Basingstoke: Palgrave, 308–28.

Smith, M.K. 2006. Community work. In *The Encyclopaedia of informal education,* www.infed.org/community/b-comwrk.htm. (accessed 19 December 2008).

Sorbonne Declaration. 1998. *Joint declaration on harmonisation of the architecture of the European higher education system.* http://www.bologna-berlin2003.de/pdf/ Sorbonne_ declaration.pdf (accessed 15 February 2009).

Stepney, P. and Ford, D. 2000. *Social work models, methods and theories: a framework for practice.* New York: Russell House Publishing.

Stevens, A. and Sullivan, D. 2001. Citizens first. *Renewal*, 9, 1, 47–54.

Taylor, C. 1992. *Multiculturalism and 'the politics of recognition'.* Princeton: Princeton University Press.

Tesluk, P. and Jacobs, R.R. 1998. Towards an integrated model of work experience. *Personnel Psychology*, 51, 2, 321–55.

Thole, W., ed. 2002a. *Grundriss Soziale Arbeit. Ein einführendes Handbuch.* Opladen: Leske und Budrich.

Thole, W. 2002b. Soziale Arbeit als Profession und Disziplin: Das sozialpädagogische Project in Praxis. Theorie, Forschung und Ausbildung – Versuch einer Standortbestimmung. In W. Thole, ed., *Grundriss Soziale Arbeit. Ein einführendes Handbuch.* Opladen: Leske und Budrich, 13–62.

Thomas, D. 1983. *The making of community work.* London: George Allen & Unwin.

Thompson, S. and Hoggett, P. 1996. Universalism, selectivism and particularism: towards a post-modern social policy. *Critical Social Policy*, 16, 21–43.

Tolan, P.H., Guerra, N.G. and Kendall, P.C. 1995. A developmental-ecological perspective on antisocial behavior in children and adolescents: toward a unified risk and intervention framework. *Journal of Consulting and Clinical Psychology*, 63, 4, 579–84.

Tomka, B. 2003. Western European welfare states in the 20th century: convergences and divergences in a long-run perspective. *International Journal of Social Welfare*, 12, 4, 249–60.

Touraine, A. 2005. *Un nouveau paradigme pour comprendre le monde d'aujourd'hui.* Paris.

Treaty on European Union, 2008. Consolidated version of the Treaty on European Union. *Official Journal of the European Union*, C 15/13 (9.5.2008).

Turner, B. ed. 1993. *Citizenship and social theory.* London: Sage.

Turner, B.S., ed. 2000. *The Blackwell companion to social theory*, 2nd edn. Malden, MA: Blackwell Publishers.

Turner, B. 2001. The erosion of citizenship. *British Journal of Sociology*, 52, 189–209.

United Nations. 2006. *Review of the first United Nations Decade for the eradication of poverty (1997–2006): Report of the Secretary-General*. New York: Economic and Social Council, UN.

Valkanova, Y. and Brehony, K. 2006. The gifts and 'contributions': Friedrich Froebel and Russian education (1850–1929). *History of Education*, 35, 2, 189–207.

Velzel, A. van. 2002. *Vraagsturing: wat kost het je?* Enschede: Wetenschapswinkel Universiteit Twente.

Visscher, S. de. 2008. *De sociaal-pedagogische betekenis van de woonomgeving voor kinderen*. Gent: Academia Press.

Volkshuisvesting, Ruimtelijke Ordening en Milieu Raad (VROM). 2006. *Stad en stijging. Sociale stijging als leidraad voor stedelijke vernieuwing*. Den Haag: VROM-raad.

Waal, V. de. 2007. *Samenspel in de buurt: burgers, professionals en beleidmakers aan zet*. Amsterdam: SWP.

Wacqaunt, L. 1999. *Les prisons de la misère*. Paris: Raisons d'Agir.

Walzer, M. 1983. *Spheres of justice: a defense of pluralism and equality*. New York: Basic Books.

Walzer, M. 1991. The idea of civil society. *Dissent*, spring, 293–304.

Wetenschappelijke Raad voor het Regeringsbeleid (WRR). 2005. *Vertrouwen in de buurt*. Amsterdam: Amsterdam University Press.

Wilken, J.P. and Hollander, D. den. 2005. *Rehabilitation and recovery*. Amsterdam: SWP.

Winter, M. de. 2000. *Beter maatschappelijk opvoeden: hoofdlijnen van een eigentijdse participatiepedagogiek*. Assen: van Gorcum.

Wistow, G., Knapp, M., Hardy, B., Forder, J., Kendall, J., and Manning R., 1996. *Social care markets: progress and prospects*. Buckingham: Open University Press.

Witteveen, W. and Klink, B. van, eds. 2002. *De sociale rechtsstaat voorbij. Twee ontwerpen voor het huis van de rechtsstaat*. Den Haag: WRR/SDU.

World Health Organisation. 1978. *Alma Ata 1978: Primary health care*. HFA Sr. No. 1.

Xu, Q. 2006. Defining international social work. *International Social Work*, 49, 6, 679–92.

Young, I.M. 1990. *Justice and the politics of difference*. Oxford: Princeton University Press.

Young, I.M. 2000. *Inclusion and democracy*. Oxford: Oxford University Press.

Yperen, T. van. 2004. Vraaggericht en effectief: tegenstelling of succesformule? Cliënt heeft geen kennis van effectieve hulpvormen. *Nederlands tijdschrift voor jeugdzorg*, 8, 1, 48–53.

Zapf, M.K. 2005. The spiritual dimension of person and environment: perspectives from social work and traditional knowledge. *International Social Work*, 48, 5, 633–42.

Zuckerman, D.M. 2000. Welfare reform in America: a clash of politics and research. *Journal of Social Issues*, 4, 587–600.

Index